AF126692

Take Me to the River

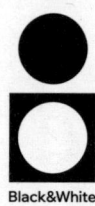

Black&White

First published in the UK in 2025 by Black & White Publishing
An imprint of Bonnier Books UK
5th Floor, HYLO, 105 Bunhill Row,
London, EC1Y 8LZ

Copyright © Vicky Allan and Jackie Kemp 2025

All rights reserved.
No part of this publication may be reproduced, stored or transmitted
in any form by any means, electronic, mechanical, photocopying or
otherwise, without the prior written permission of the publisher.

The right of Vicky Allan and Jackie Kemp to be identified as Author
of this work has been asserted by them in accordance with the
Copyright, Designs and Patents Act, 1988.

The publisher has made every reasonable effort to contact copyright holders
of extracts used in this book. Any errors are inadvertent and anyone who for any
reason has not been contacted is invited to write to the publisher so that a full
acknowledgement can be made in subsequent editions of this work.

A CIP catalogue record for this book is available from the British Library.

ISBN: 978 1 78530 623 5

1 3 5 7 9 10 8 6 4 2

Typeset by Tonje Hefte / IDSUK (Data Connection) Ltd
Printed and bound in Great Britain by Clays Ltd, Elcograf S.p.A.

The authorised representative in the EEA is Bonnier Books UK (Ireland) Limited.
Registered office address: Floor 3, Block 3, Miesian Plaza, Dublin 2, D02 Y754, Ireland
compliance@bonnierbooks.ie

www.bonnierbooks.co.uk

Take Me to the River

More than 100 authors on bathing in nature

Vicky Allan and
Jackie Kemp

Black&White

'This plunge into the cold water of a mountain pool seems for a brief moment to disintegrate the very self; it is not to be borne: one is lost: stricken: annihilated. Then life pours back.'

— NAN SHEPHERD, *The Living Mountain*[1]

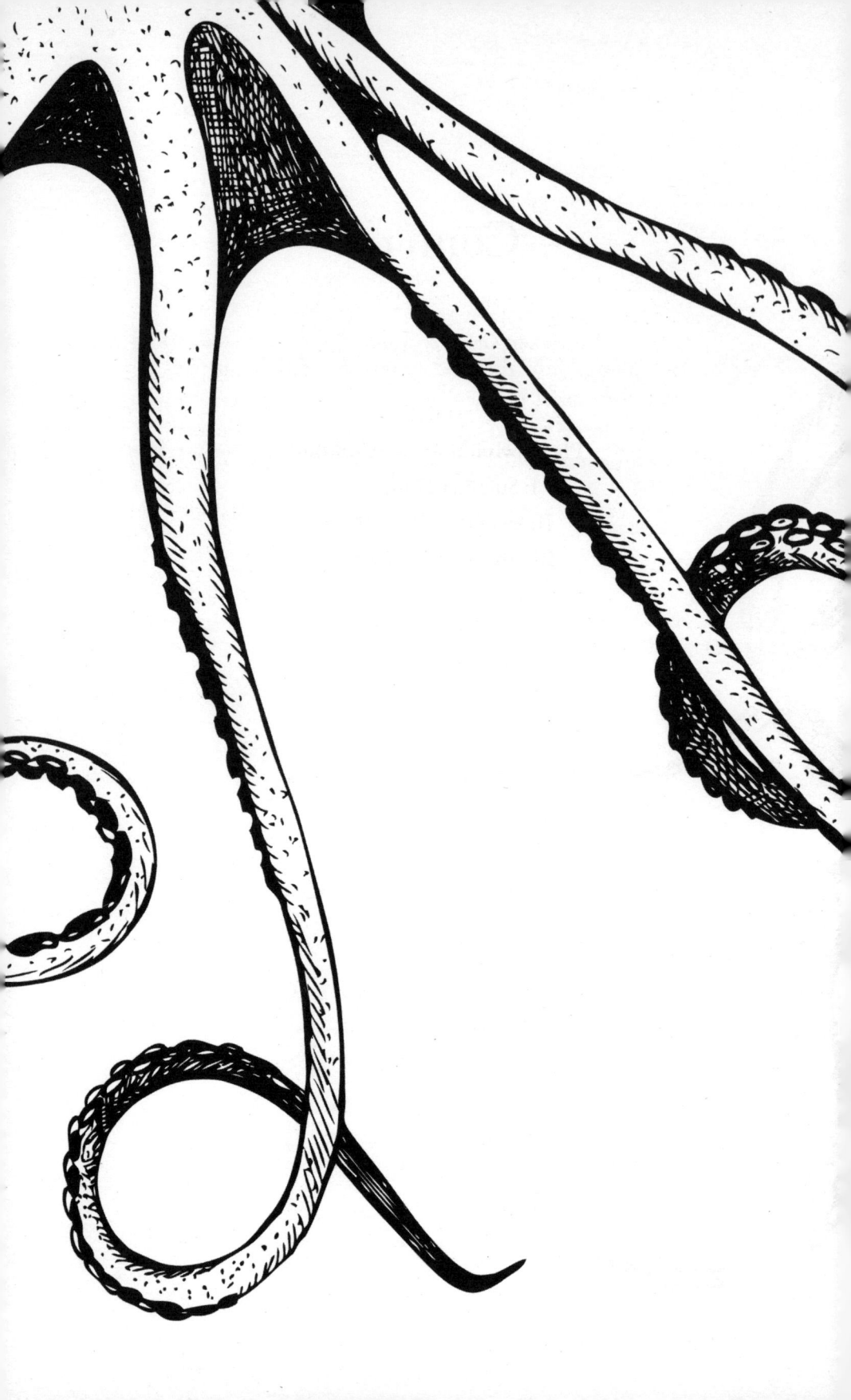

Contents

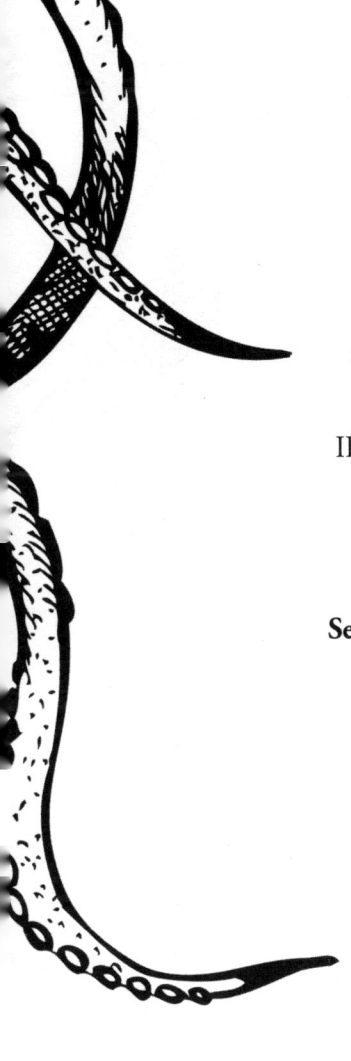

An Ocean of Words   xi

ONE

Play: Swimming and Childhood

I: Summer Holidays   5

II: Swimming Lessons   23

III: The Right to Swim   31

IV: Parents on the Edge   43

V: Adventure   58

VI: Adults at Play   70

TWO

Scary: Monsters and Marvels

I: See Monsters   85

II: Marvellous Sea Creatures   97

III: Monsters Are Us   104

THREE

Sensation: Swimming and Desire

I: Feeling Water   121

II: Erotic Encounters   127

III: Old Times   146

IV: The Male Gaze   152

V: Sexy Beasts   160

VI: Free From the Gaze   164

FOUR

Epic: Great Swims

I: Cold Waters, Cold Wars 175

II: Strong Swimmers 189

III: Ancients   206

IV: Alongside Swim Heroes 213

V: Lost 220

FIVE

Well: The Cold Water Cure

I: Recovery   237

II: The Doctor's Line   248

III: Taking the Waters   256

IV: Literally Wild   267

V: Rediscovery   270

SIX

Deep: Swimming and Symbolism

I: Océanique   281

II: The Sea as Mother   296

III: Underworlds   304

IV: The Power of Nature   316

V: Journey's end   325

Finding Ourselves   339

Reading List   343

Acknowledgements   354

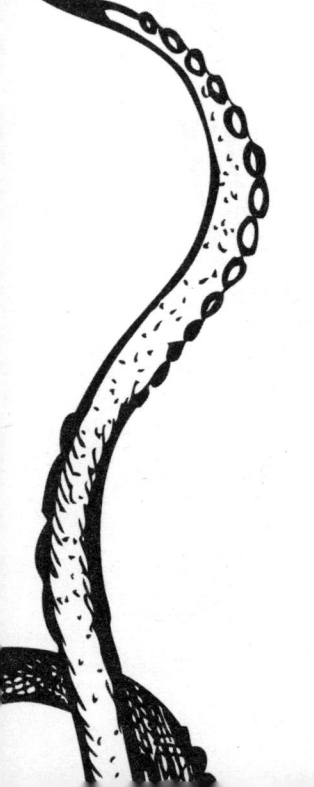

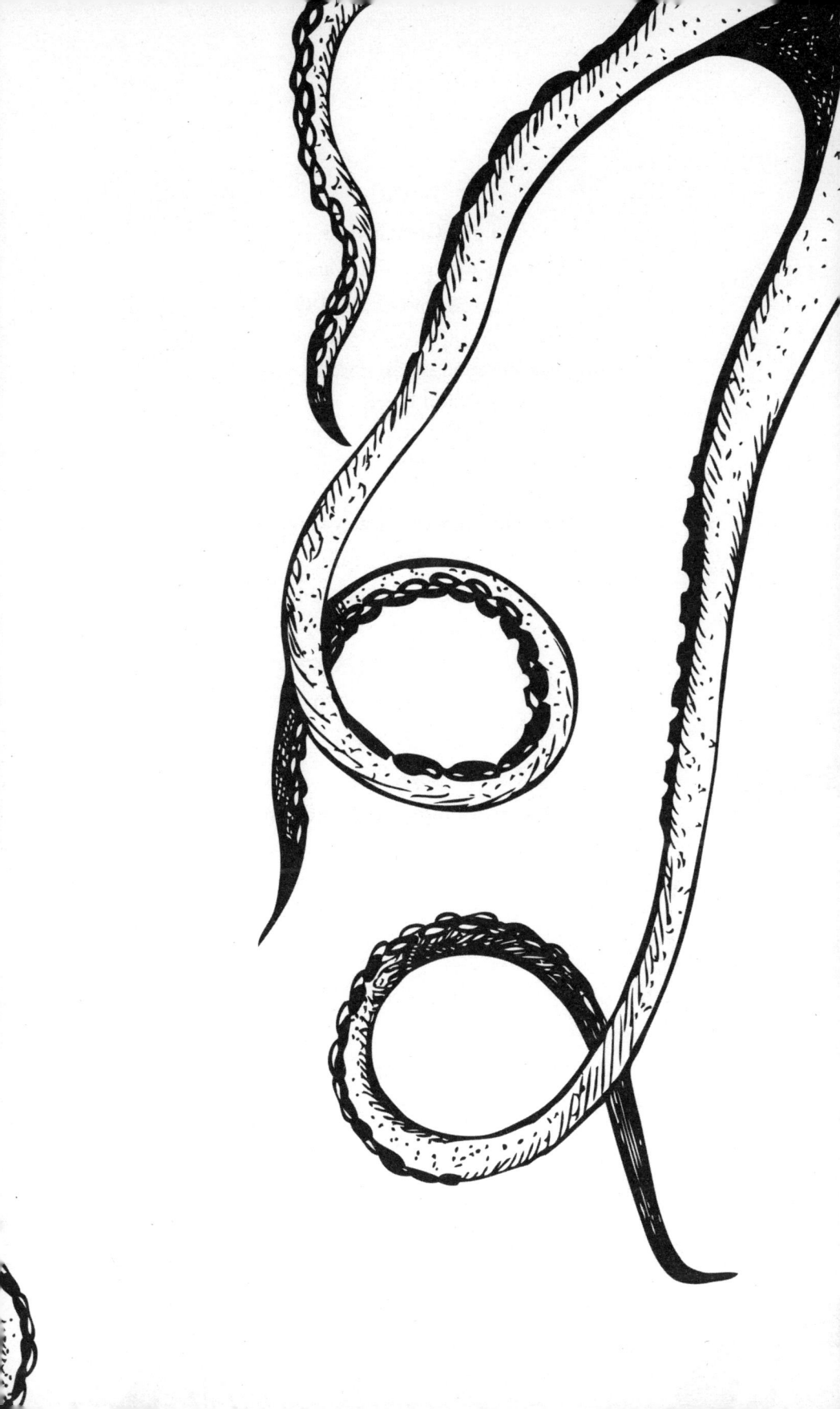

Something had pestered me so much
I thought my heart would break
I mean, the mechanical part.
I went down in the afternoon
to the sea
which held me, until I grew easy.

— MARY OLIVER,
from 'Swimming, One Day in August'[2]

An Ocean of Words

We talked about books before we ever swam together. The conversation would often take a long, deep dive into the entangled literary world of words. We were members of a book group in Leith before either of us joined any swim group. Friday nights over glasses of wine, putting the world to rights.

So it was natural that when we both started swimming that the chat would turn to our favourite watery scenes in books. 'Have you read Iris Murdoch's, *The Sea, The Sea*? That incredible scene where the character is gazing down into the water and sees a monster rising . . .'

'What about Mark Twain?'

'And Nan Shepherd's line about a plunge into a mountain pool, that phrase about life pouring back. It's like the full cold water journey in a couple of sentences.'

'And Mary Oliver's poem where she says the sea held her "until I grew easy"?'

That was how this book began. It became a kind of swim journey, taken partly in bodies of water – the North Sea, where we plunged off Portobello town beach, to the wintry mirror of Loch Torridon, in Wester Ross where Jackie is now based, and where we bounced ideas around a studio office. But it also took us to the walnut-and-leather desked reading rooms of the National Library of Scotland. Some of the books we looked through there — like a nineteenth-century translation of Egyptian papyrus — didn't make the final cut, but it was a pleasure to turn the pages of rare volumes like this.

What we also shared was a feeling that wild swimming is a way of being in nature. There's much debate around the use of the term, and that word 'wild', but what it expresses, and has done since Roger Deakin first coined it, is an immersion in natural waters, and all the marvellous life they support. You take off your clothes — or most of them — leave the phone behind and submerge. You move your body to accommodate yourself to a different element. You are in nature, not an observer or an extractor; you are part of it. You have that 'frog's eye' view of the world, the perspective that Deakin wrote about.

A seal pops a whiskery face up, metres away. A dark brown guillemot floats by, seemingly regarding the human head as just another piece of flotsam.

In the sea or the lake or the river you can play. You can engage with other beings — maybe humans, maybe not.

We found ourselves sharing quotes about the wonders of that aquatic life.

We talked about American ichthyologist, Eugenie Clark, popularly known as the shark lady, who in her old age said: 'Everything I've done, I've enjoyed doing. I've had five husbands, four children. I've done it all, but mainly I've enjoyed studying fish and being underwater with them, being in their natural habitat, looking at the fish and the fish looking at me.'

So many of the passages we shared with each other were, we began to notice, a form of nature writing. They are about the human body, yes, and the act of swimming, but they are also about what we swim in, and alongside.

This book is a dive in and out of different minds and bodies, through diverse watery experiences, as well as a journey through our own swimming and reading lives. We hope you enjoy taking a plunge.

Jackie Kemp and Vicky Allan

Throughout the book we introduce and comment on the extracts we have chosen for this anthology, sometimes together, and sometimes with personal stories. In these instances, we have left a little symbol to let you know who is talking.

Vicky's narrative is marked with a starfish.

Jackie's narrative is marked with a sea shell.

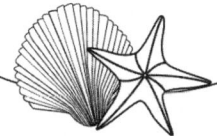

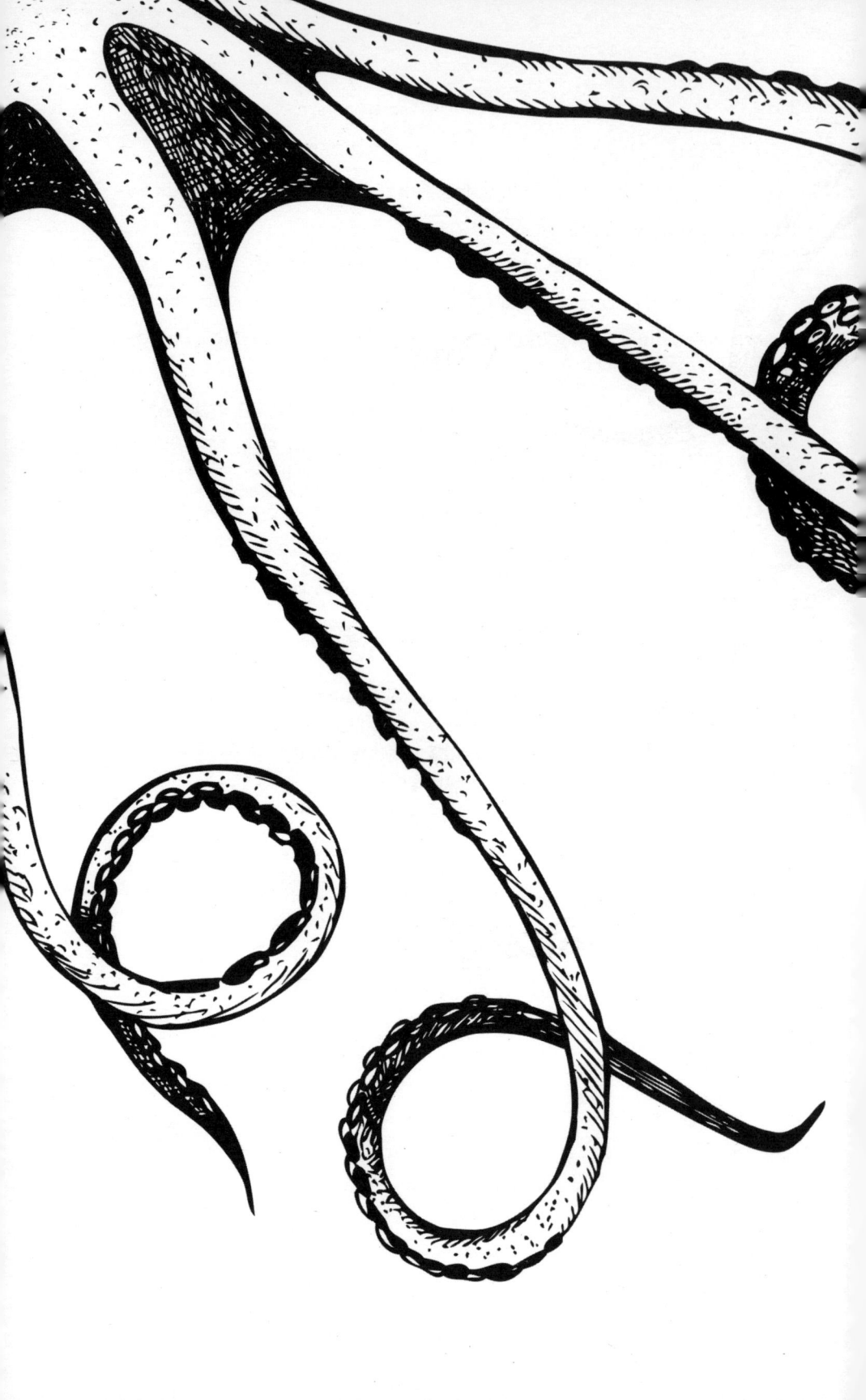

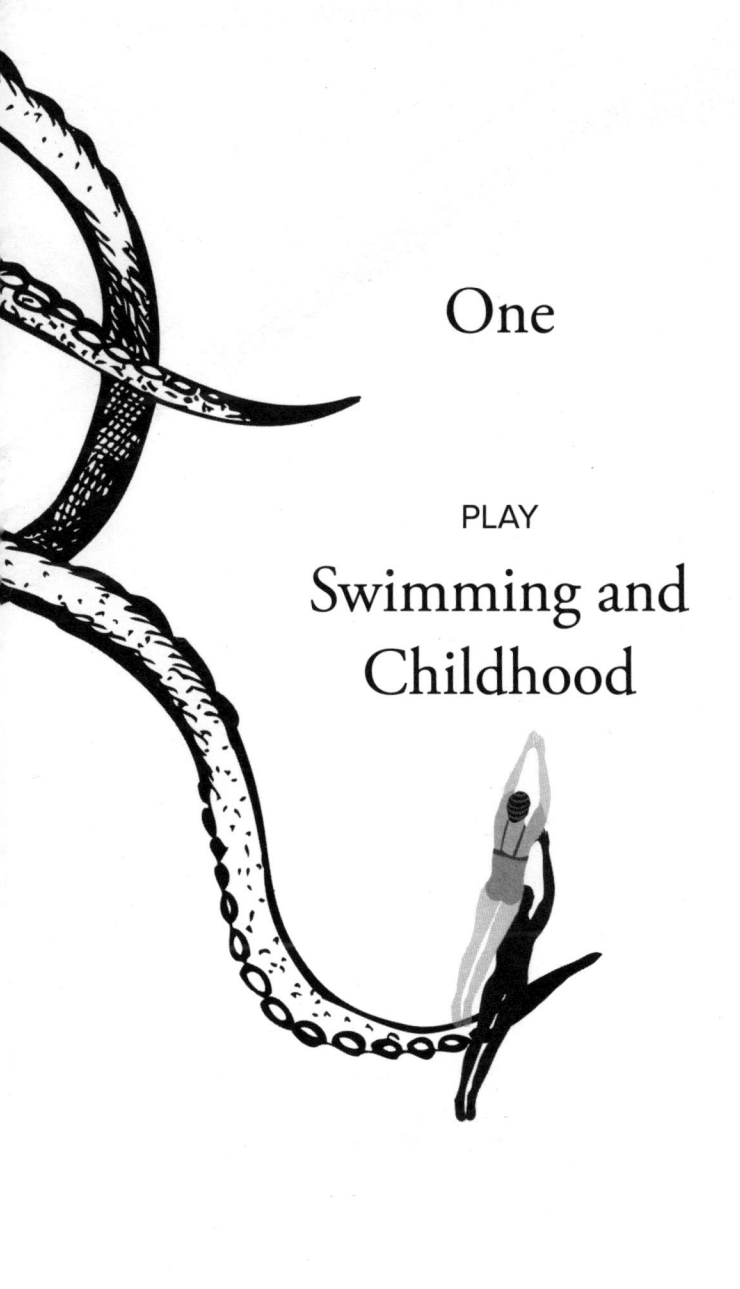

One

PLAY

Swimming and Childhood

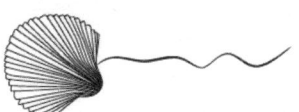

I CAN STILL RECALL THE feel of the scratchy towel that enveloped me as I emerged from the North Sea into my mother's arms as a child in Scotland. After being rubbed down, my sister and I would run across the windblown sand to get the blood back into our reddened limbs. On picnics in the hills, we pootered about in peaty rivers, building dams with my father.

And on the beach with my own kids, and their friends, we built not just sandcastles but sand masterpieces – towers of stones, mermaids with seaweed hair, sleeping elephants, and once, the huge, sandalled foot of Jesus. The fruit of our artistic labours was soon washed away – but the memories remain.

Robert Burns wrote in *Auld Lang Syne*: 'We twa hae paiddled i' the burn fae mornin sun til dine/ But the seas between us baith hae roared sin auld lang syne.' Those play-filled hours are the basis for friendships that survive time and distance.

People come back to the shore as parents, aunties and uncles, or just as adults keen to reconnect with those simple pleasures. But swimming is not all joy – V. S. Naipaul's *A House for Mr Biswas* includes an episode when a family's seaside experience is painfully different from the picture painted in children's books of the time. Richard Wright's horror at the swimming hole was inspired by real incidents of racism over the right to swim.

CHAPTER I

Summer Holidays

MY OWN SUMMER HOLIDAYS WERE pretty uneventful. The highlight was generally a trip to the well-stocked children's section of a municipal library. But in my imagination, I travelled far and had many adventures. Arthur Ransome's stories, based on his own childhood trips to the English Lakes in the late nineteenth century, became the ur-holidays – the ones to measure all others by. The children in his books had an extraordinary degree of freedom and agency. Their untrammelled lives, in and out of the water, escaping adult control, were punctuated by simple but hearty meals, as in this excerpt.

In the introduction to *Swallows and Amazons*, Ransome wrote:

I have often been asked how I came to write *Swallows and Amazons*. The answer is that it had its beginnings long, long ago when, as children, my brother, my sisters and I spent most of our holidays on a farm north of Coniston. We played in or on the lake or in the hills above it, finding friends in the farmers and shepherds and charcoal-burners whose smoke rose from the coppice woods along the shore. We adored the place. Coming to it, we used to rush down to the lake, dip our hands in and wish, as if we had just seen the new moon. Going away from it, we were half drowned in tears. While away from it, as children and grown-ups, we dreamt about it. No matter where I was, wandering about the world, I used at night to look for the North Star and, in my mind's eye, could see the beloved skyline of great hills beneath it.

The four Walker siblings ask for parental permission to camp alone on an island for their entire school holiday. Their mother puts this request to their absent father by letter. The book opens with seven-year-old Roger tacking across the field holding the telegram reply. It reads cryptically 'IF DUFFERS WILL DROWN' – duffers being a naval term for a bad sailor. The sensitive Titty (short for Tatiana) correctly interprets this as a challenge to their mother: 'Mummy doesn't think we are duffers.'

'Titty, privately, was being a cormorant.'
Swallows and Amazons by Arthur Ransome[3]

'You're to swim as well as splash,' said Mate Susan.

'Aye, aye, sir,' said Roger. He crouched in the water with only his head out. That, at least, felt very like swimming. John and Susan swam races, first one way, and then the other. Titty, privately, was being a cormorant. This was not the sort of thing that she could very well talk of to John or Susan until she was sure that it was a success. So she said nothing about it. But she had seen that there were lots of minnows in the shallow water close to the shore. Perhaps there would be bigger ones further out, like the fish the cormorants had been catching yesterday. She watched them carefully. The way they did it was to swim quietly and then suddenly to dive under water, humping their backs, keeping their wings close together, and going under head first. She tried, but she found that unless she used her arms, she did not get under water at all. Even when she used her arms she could not get right under without a long, splashing struggle on the surface.

'Why do you wave your legs in the air, Titty?' Roger asked after one of these dives. It was too true. Titty herself knew that long after she had put her head under and was swimming downwards as hard as she could her legs were kicking out of the water altogether. She went further out, to be nearer the fish, and further from Roger. At last she found the trick of turning her hands so that her arm strokes pulled her down. She found that she could open her eyes easily enough, but that it was like trying to see in a bright green fog. There were no fish to be seen in it. With a great effort, she got right down to the bottom. Still there were no fish. She came up puffing, then dived again and again. It was no good. She picked a stone off the bottom to make sure that she had really been there, and came to the top again in a hurry, spluttering and out of breath. There was no doubt about it. The fish could see her coming, and could swim faster than she could. There was nothing for it but fishing rods. She swam in towards the beach holding her stone.

'What have you got?' said Roger.

'A stone,' said Titty. 'I got it off the bottom.'

'What sort of a stone?'

'Probably a pearl. Let's be pearl-divers.'

Cormorants were forgotten, and the able-seaman and the boy were pearl-divers in a moment . . .

'Come on, Roger,' said Captain John, let's see you swim with both feet on the bottom . . . 'Try swimming on your back,' said John.

'Can't,' said Roger.

'It's easy. Stand like this in the water, leaning back. Then put your ears under.'

Roger leant back.

'Ears right under,' said John.

'They are,' said Roger.

Even as he said it, there was a wild splashing, and Roger disappeared. He was up again at once, spluttering.

'I couldn't keep my feet on the bottom,' he said. They came up of themselves.

'I knew they would,' said John. 'If you hadn't doubled up you'd have floated.'

Titty was swimming round them like a dog, paddling with her arms and legs, not in pairs, but one after another. 'Try it again, Roger,' she said.

'I'll put a hand under the back of your neck so that your mouth won't go under,' said John.

Roger leant back once more, and rested his head on John's hand. He pressed his ears under, and again his feet floated up.

Kick,' said John. 'Kick like a frog. Kick again. You're swimming. Well done.'

'You really did swim on your back,' said Titty, as Roger struggled to his feet again.

'I know I did,' said Roger. Watch now.' He leant back towards the shore, put his ears under, and kicked hard. He got three good kicks in before he ran aground. He had swum three yards at least. But Mate Susan had not seen him. She had just had a few minutes' good hard swim, and then had run up to the camp again to dry and dress, and see to her fire and the kettle at the same time. There were eggs to boil, and bread and butter to cut. The mate's job is not an easy one, with a hungry crew to feed. Roger looked round for her, splashed out of the water, and ran, prancing, up to the camp to tell her that he had swum on his back.

'Did you really swim?' said the mate.

'Aye, aye, sir,' said the boy. 'Three kicks, not touching anything.

Come down, and I'll show you.'

'Can't now,' said the mate. 'You dry yourself and help to get the breakfast.'

~

TOVE JANSSON ACHIEVED INTERNATIONAL FAME for her children's series, the Moomins. But her novel *The Summer Book*, first published in 1972, is much loved for its tender portrayal of the relationship between a grandmother and her six-year-old granddaughter as they spend summer together on a tiny island in Finland.

'You let go of everything and just dive.'
The Summer Book by Tove Jansson
(translated from Swedish by Thomas Teal)[4]

The Morning Swim
It was an early, very warm morning in July, and it had rained during the night. The bare granite steamed, the moss and crevices were drenched with moisture, and all the colours everywhere had deepened. Below the veranda, the vegetation in the morning shade was like a rainforest of lush, evil leaves and flowers, which she had to be careful not to break as she searched. She held one hand in front of her mouth and was constantly afraid of losing her balance.

'What are you doing?' asked little Sophia.

'Nothing,' her grandmother answered. 'That is to say,' she added angrily, 'I'm looking for my false teeth.'

The child came down from the veranda. 'Where did you lose them?' she asked.

'Here,' said her grandmother. 'I was standing right there and they fell somewhere in the peonies.'

They looked together.

'Let me,' Sophia said. 'You can hardly walk. Move over.'

She dived beneath the flowering roof of the garden and crept among green stalks and stems. It was pretty and mysterious down on the soft black earth. And there were the teeth, white and pink, a whole mouthful of old teeth.

'I've got them!' the child cried, and stood up. 'Put them in.'

'But you can't watch,' Grandmother said. 'That's private.'

Sophia held the teeth behind her back.

'I want to watch,' she said.

So Grandmother put the teeth in, with a smacking noise. They went in very easily. It had really hardly been worth mentioning.

'When are you going to die?' the child asked.

And Grandmother answered, 'Soon. But that is not the least concern of yours.'

'Why?' her grandchild asked.

She didn't answer. She walked out on the rock and on towards the ravine.

'We're not allowed out there!' Sophia screamed.

'I know,' the old woman answered disdainfully. 'Your father won't let either one of us go out to the ravine, but we're going anyway, because your father is asleep and he won't know.'

They walked across the granite. The moss was slippery. The sun had come up a good way now, and everything was steaming. The whole island was covered with a bright haze. It was very pretty.

'Will they dig a hole?' asked the child amiably.

'Yes,' she said. 'A big hole.' And she added, insidiously, 'Big enough for all of us.'

'How come?' the child asked.

They walked on towards the point.

'I've never been this far before,' Sophia said. 'Have you? '

'No,' her grandmother said.

They walked all the way out onto the little promontory, where the rock descended into the water in water terraces that became fainter and fainter until there was total darkness. Each step down was edged with a light green seaweed fringe that swayed back and forth with the movement of the sea.

'I want to go swimming,' the child said. She waited for opposition, but none came. So she took off her clothes, slowly and nervously. She glanced at her grandmother – you can't depend on people who just let things happen. She put her legs in the water.

'It's cold,' she said.

'Of course it's cold,' the old woman said, her thoughts somewhere else. 'What did you expect?'

The child slid in up to her waist and waited anxiously.

'Swim,' her grandmother said. 'You can swim.'

It's deep, Sophia thought. She forgets I've never swum in deep water unless somebody was with me. And she climbed out again and sat down on the rock.

'It's going to be a nice day today,' she declared.

The sun had climbed higher. The whole island, and the sea, were glistening. The air seemed very light.

'I can dive,' Sophia said. 'Do you know what it feels like when you dive?'

'Of course I do,' her grandmother said. 'You can feel the seaweed against your legs. It's brown, and the water's clear, lighter towards the top, with lots of bubbles. And you glide. You hold your breath and glide and turn and come up, let yourself rise and breathe out. And then you float. Just float.'

'And all the time with your eyes open,' Sophia said.

'Naturally. People don't dive with their eyes shut.'

'Do you believe I can dive without me showing you?' the child asked.

'Yes, of course,' Grandmother said. 'Now get dressed. We can get back before he wakes up.'

The first weariness came closer. When we get home, she thought, when we get back I think I'll take a little nap. And I must remember to tell him this child is still afraid of deep water.

~

NOT EVERY CHILD LONGS FOR the summer holidays to go on forever. In an essay originally published in 2011 in *The New Yorker*, David Sedaris recalls the 'chemical baths' of country club swimming pools in North Carolina in the 1960s. Pushed into the swim team, David felt bruised by his father's admiration for the boy who always won.

'In retrospect, I was never an awful swimmer, just average.'
'Memory Laps' by David Sedaris[5]

On a hot, windless afternoon you could probably smell them from an equal distance. Chlorine pits is what they were. Chemical baths. In the deep end my sisters and I would dive for nickels. Toss one in and by the time we reached it half of Jefferson's face would be eaten away. Come lunchtime, we'd line up at the snack bar, our hair the texture of cotton candy, our small, burning eyes like little cranberries.

I took my lessons in June of 1966, the first year of our membership.

By the following summer, I was on the swim team. This sounds like an accomplishment, but I believe that in 1967 anyone could be on the Raleigh Country Club team. All you had to do was show up and wear an orange Speedo.

Before my first practice, I put swimming in the same category as walking and riding a bike: things one did to get from place to place. I never thought of how well I was doing them. It was only in competing that an activity became fraught and self-conscious. More accurately, it was only in competing with boys. I was fine against girls, especially if they were younger than me. Younger than me and physically challenged was even better. Give me a female opponent with a first-grade education and a leg brace, and I would churn that water like a speedboat. When it came to winning, I never split hairs.

Most of my ribbons were for good sportsmanship, a backhanded compliment if ever there was one. As the starting gun was raised, I would look at my competitors twitching at their places. Parents would shout their boozy encouragement from the sidelines, and it would occur to me that one of us would have to lose, that I could do that for these people. For, whether I placed or came in last, all I ultimately felt was relief. The race was over, and now I could go home. Then the next meet would be announced, and it would start again: the sleepless nights, the stomach aches, a crippling and all-encompassing sense of doom. My sisters Lisa and Gretchen were on the team as well, but I don't think it bothered them as much. For me, every meet day was the same. "Mom"—this said with a groan, like someone calling out from beneath a boulder—"I don't feel too good. Maybe we should . . ."

"Oh, no you don't."

If I had been trying to get out of school, she'd have at least allowed me to plead my case, but then she had no presence at school. At the club she was front and center, laughing it up with Ike at the bar and with the girls in the restaurant beside the putting green. Once summer got going, we'd spend all day at the pool, us swimming and her broasting on one of the deck chairs. Every so often, she'd go into the water to cool off, but she didn't know how to swim and didn't trust us not to drag her under. So she'd sit waist-deep in the kiddie pool, dropping her cigarette ash onto the wet pavement and dissolving it with her finger.

There was a good-sized group of women like her, and they were united in their desire to be left alone. Run to your mother with a complaint, and before she could speak one of the others would say, "Oh, come on now. Let's not be a tattletale," or, "You would have lost that tooth anyway. Now get back into the water." I think of them in that terrible heat, no umbrellas, just sunglasses and bottles of tanning oil that left them smelling like coconuts.

The pool was a land of women and children until swim meets, which usually started at six. Then drinks would be ordered and the dads would arrive. For most of the fathers, this was just one more thing they had to turn up for. Their son was likely on his school's football or basketball team. Maybe he played baseball as well. For my dad, though, this was it, and, the way I saw it, he should have been grateful. Look at all the time my fear of sports was affording him—weekends and evenings free.

In retrospect, I was never an awful swimmer, just average. I'd come in third sometimes, and once or twice, if I was part of a relay team, we'd place first, though I could hardly take credit. Occasionally, we'd have intra-club races, us against us, and in those, as in the larger meets, the star was a boy named Greg Sakas, who was my size but a few years younger, with pale-yellow hair and legs no thicker than jumper cables. "God, that Greg Sakas, did you see him go?" my father said on the way home from my first meet. "Man alive, that kid is faaaantastic."

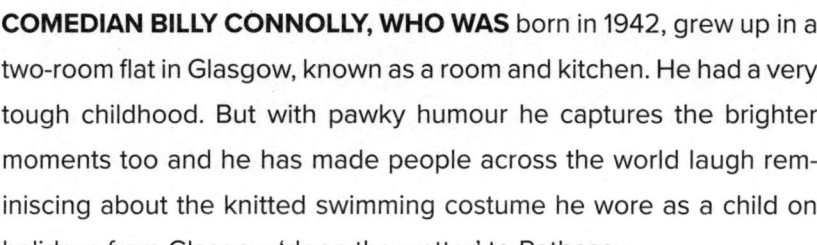

COMEDIAN BILLY CONNOLLY, WHO WAS born in 1942, grew up in a two-room flat in Glasgow, known as a room and kitchen. He had a very tough childhood. But with pawky humour he captures the brighter moments too and he has made people across the world laugh reminiscing about the knitted swimming costume he wore as a child on holidays from Glasgow 'doon the watter' to Rothesay.

'There was a lovely innocence about it all.'
Made in Scotland: My Grand Adventures in a Wee Country by Billy Connolly[6]

My main great childhood experiences of Scotland outside of Glasgow came each July, when my father took Florence and me on holiday to Rothesay on the Isle of Bute. In the second fortnight in July, the factories would shut down and Glasgow would just empty out as everybody went on holiday down the Clyde. They used to call it the Glasgow Fair holidays. The whole city would have two weeks off and go away, and when we came back from our holidays it would be Paisley's turn.

It was all such an amazing, exciting ritual. We would get the train out of Glasgow Central and it would be jammed with hundreds of people and their suitcases, and children running around, laughing and shouting. When we arrived at Wemyss Bay station, everybody would spew out of the train on to the platform and march down a concrete walkway to the ferry stop like a huge invading army. It was brilliant to see the Clyde and know we were about to sail across it. My father would be saying, 'C'mon, Billy, keep up!' as he strode along, and Florence and I would get more and more carried away with it all.

A ferry would be sitting waiting with its wooden gangway coming down onto the pier, and we'd all pour on. I would be so excited running up the gangway: 'Woah! Here we go!' The ferries were these great paddle steamers, and I can remember their names as if it were yesterday: the *Jeanie Deans*. The *Queen Mary II*. The *Caledonia*. The *Duchess of Montrose*. The *Waverley*. The one I remember best is the *Marchioness of Breadalbane*. We always seemed to get that one.

When you got on the ferry, the first thing you would hear would be the fiddling and the accordions as two guys and a woman sang songs on the boat. They would sing tunes like 'The Song of the Clyde':

Oh, the River Clyde, the wonderful Clyde,
The name of it thrills me and fills me with pride
And I'm satisfied, whate'er may betide,
The sweetest of songs is the Song of the Clyde.

The men would sing the song and the woman would go about the ferry with a velvet bag, looking for donations. There was a lovely innocence about it all: singing songs about your country and going down the Clyde for the Glasgow Fair holiday. Everybody was going away at the same time so you'd see all your school friends running around the boat. You would go down to the ferry's engine room to see the paddle steamer engines, with their great huge pistons rolling away. There was a sweetie shop on board where, if you were lucky, your parents would buy you lemonade.

You would sail down the Clyde and the view on the bank either side was like nothing you were used to in Glasgow. It was all forests and gold-coloured harvest fields, what the Scots call hairst fields. There is a lovely bit of Scottish verse about it:

O yellow lie the hairst fields
along the banks o' Clyde
They are the bonniest hairst fields
that ever was beside.

All we had done was step off a train but we had gone from the world
we knew into a completely new one. You would meet people that you
knew from Glasgow and you wouldn't recognise them because they had
their good clothes on. You were used to seeing them in overalls and flat
caps but here they were in smart shirts with sleeves rolled up, striding
along with their wife and family. You wouldn't know them and they
would have to remind you who they were . . .

The second fortnight in July is traditionally a pretty rainy time of
year – as I've always said, there are two seasons in Scotland: June and
Winter – so we'd often be sitting in the pouring rain singing those songs.
I have photographs of Flo and me standing on the beach in trench coats
and wellies holding buckets and spades in a downpour. Glaswegians of
my age have all got those photos . . .

The pelting rain on holiday didn't stop Florence and me swimming
in the sea in our swimming costumes. My costume was a monstrosity
that still traumatises me to this day. My aunt had knitted it for me, which
meant that it was made of wool and had no elastic. I had to wear a belt
with it. It had a wee pocket knitted in it. I wondered for years what I
was supposed to keep in there. Maybe four pennies for the telephone in
case I was drowning. It was dark blue but it turned brown in the water,
which was very unfortunate. It would look like a brown kilt that had
been in a hurricane. There was an Italian boy in my class at school called
Nino Manibli, who was very stylish. He had the best swimming costume
you ever saw, all red-and-white satin with laces up both sides, and there

17

was I, in blue-turning-brown-wool with a belt. I used to fantasise about murdering Nino in his bed to steal his costume.

Florence and I would swim at Rothesay beach and beneath the water my costume would transform into a drogue parachute. The crotch would be down around my knees, as if I was being pursued by a dark blue nappy. It would slow me down: I would swim my hardest and go nowhere. When I came out of the water, I had to grab the back of my costume and pull it back in order to pull the front up and stop my family jewels flopping out and scaring the other children on the beach. The costume would be running like a tap and it would look as if I was peeing myself on the sand. After I'd been swimming, it would take two weeks to dry out.

I wasn't the only guy with a knitted costume, though. They were a big thing. Sometimes we would swim in the swimming pool in Rothesay. It had a café underneath it with windows into the pool and you could see the people's legs. So, there would be headless people swimming, flailing around, trying to keep their costume on, with the crotch flapping around their ankles, while people were trying to eat their scones:

Mummy, Mummy, what's that?

Look away! Look away, Lucinda! Cover your eyes! I think that man is having a fit! And that might be a haemorrhoid!

Our two weeks in Rothesay would be over in no time and we'd be back at the harbour waiting for the ferry home. The incoming Paisley holidaymakers would all come down the gangway and my father would tell Florence and me, 'Go and give your buckets and spades away.' We'd go up to children coming off the boat and give them to them, and off they'd go on holiday with our buckets and spades.

NOEL STREATFEILD IS MOST FAMOUS for the children's classic *Ballet Shoes*, published in 1936, but she wrote many other books for children, often about the struggles of middle-class families like her own.

Anyone who has ever felt part of the 'squeezed middle' might identify with this account of penny-pinching summer holidays, trapping young teenagers in boring country cottages, in Streatfeild's lightly fictionalised memoir. But they too had their ur-holiday – one when the sun shone and they socialised with local teens.

'Daddy thinks it more fun when it is cold and rough.'

A Vicarage Family by Noel Streatfeild[7]

St Margaret's remained for always a mountain-top of a holiday; one by which all others could be measured. Afterwards all the family knew what was meant by 'Nearly as good as St Margaret's Bay'. Every year in the spring, the children's father would look up from a letter and announce as if it was an award the name of some minute village in Wales, Devonshire, Essex, Derbyshire or wherever he had rented for the month of August. Later snippets of information would come out. First, the historical background of the place to be visited and later, bits culled from tourist guides. 'The part of Essex where we are staying is called "Poppy-land". In North Wales on Sunday choirs sing hymns on the beach. In Derbyshire, they eat cheese with cake.'

To the children's father, whose day started at seven, except on Sundays, Saints' days and special occasions, when he was never up later than six; who seldom got to bed before two in the morning; who never sat down between these hours except in church, at a meeting or for hurried meals; who went everywhere on foot so that any-one could waylay him; that distant holiday must have looked an oasis indeed. But his family, though they had enjoyed the holiday when they were small, were now out-growing it. They never said so in so many words, but there were occasional slips. After the holiday spent in an exceptionally dreary house on a bleak spot on the Essex Coast Dick was heard to say: 'Isn't it glorious to be home after that awful Poppy-land!' And after the Derbyshire holiday Isobel, swallowing some medicine, Isabel remarked: 'It's nearly as nasty as Derbyshire.'

All such slips were either laughed off or crushed as heresy by the children's mother who saw all too clearly the gap widening between the children's father's dream family built on his boyhood home and his real family. No doubt family holidays when he was a boy had been fun, for there was less shortage of money. But no one could blame his children if they got quarrelsome or bored in the let's-get-away-from-it-all houses far from anywhere which was all they could afford. For, contrary to belief, Augusts in those days were just as wet as they are now.

During the Derbyshire August, it rained every day and the only dry spot was a waterfall the family had tramped miles to see. The cheap houses were totally unfitted with amusements indoors for a growing family, for they seldom had any books – and never any games. Yet somehow, however depressing the holiday, the children's mother helped to keep the myth going that a jolly holiday was being enjoyed by all, for otherwise it would be all too easy for her husband to say: 'I don't think I need a holiday this year.'

There were many reasons why St Margaret's Bay was a landmark holiday. First, the weather was kind, it was an exceptionally hot, dry summer. This made bathing, always the high spot of their father's holiday, able to be enjoyed by his children, which in wet summers it never was.

'I can just see my father and Uncle Jim and all the other uncles swimming half-way to France,' John had told Victoria as, with blue faces and chattering teeth after a bathe, they ate buns on an icy beach. I think summer must have been warmer then.'

It was the North Wales year. Victoria looked at her father, also blue of face, coming out from behind the rock he had used as a dressing room. 'I bet you it wasn't, Daddy thinks it more fun when it is cold and rough.' And it was true for at that moment her father, blowing on his fingers which were white where the circulation had stopped, said: 'I think that's the best bathe we've had. Wouldn't it be fun, if it doesn't rain, if we came down again this afternoon for the tide will be in, and the waves should be much bigger.'

'Have a bun, darling,' the children's mother said. I think one bathe is enough and if it keeps fine I thought we would go blackberrying.' But at Margaret's Bay bathing was a real joy, so there was no need to pretend, and no excuses had to be found why there should not be a second bathe.

~

THE WAY CHILDREN PLAY AT the beach feels timeless. 'At the Bay', written in 1921, is a long short story by Katherine Mansfield, set in a beach resort, a summer colony inhabited during the day only by women and children, while the men go back into town each day to work.

'As for Lottie, she liked to be left to go in her own way.'
'At the Bay' by Katherine Mansfield[8]

As the morning lengthened whole parties appeared over the sand-hills and came down on the beach to bathe. It was understood that at eleven o'clock the women and children of the summer colony had the sea to themselves. First the women undressed, pulled on their bathing dresses and covered their heads in hideous caps like sponge bags; then the children were unbuttoned. The beach was strewn with little heaps of clothes and shoes; the big summer hats, with stones on them to keep them from blowing away, looked like immense shells. It was strange that even the sea seemed to sound differently when all those leaping, laughing figures ran into the waves. Old Mrs. Fairfield, in a lilac cotton dress and a black hat tied under the chin, gathered her little brood and got them ready. The little Trout boys whipped their shirts over their heads, and away the five sped, while their grandma sat with one hand in her knitting-bag ready to draw out the ball of wool when she was satisfied they were safely in.

The firm compact little girls were not half so brave as the tender, delicate-looking boys. Pip and Rags, shivering, crouching down, slapping the water, never hesitated. But Isabel, who could swim twelve strokes, and Kezia, who could nearly swim eight, only followed on the strict understanding they were not to be splashed. As for Lottie, she didn't follow at all. She liked to be left to go in her own way, please. And that way was to sit down at the edge of the water, her legs straight, her knees pressed together, and to make vague motions with her arms as if she expected to be wafted out to sea. But when a bigger wave than usual, an old whiskery one, came lolloping along in her direction, she scrambled to her feet with a face of horror and flew up the beach again.

CHAPTER II

Swimming Lessons

THE FIRST TIME YOU LIFT your feet off the bottom and manage to move forward is a big moment. Most of us learn in swimming pools, with the help of instructors or parents, but the nineteenth-century environmentalist John Muir taught himself to swim by copying the frogs, in a pond near his home.

We have Muir to thank for America's National Parks, which he helped to found. Born in Scotland, John emigrated at the age of eleven to the USA with his family to the state of Wisconsin, sometimes known as 'the land of 10,000 lakes'. As a teenager, Muir found respite from life with his domineering father in nature, both on land and in the water.

'Go to the frogs and they will give you all the lessons you need.'
The Story of My Boyhood and Youth by John Muir[9]

One hot summer day Father told us that we ought to learn to swim. This was one of the most interesting suggestions he had ever offered, but precious little time was allowed for trips to the lake, and he seldom tried to show us how. 'Go to the frogs,' he said, 'and they will give you all the lessons you need. Watch their arms and legs and see how smoothly they kick themselves along and dive and come up. When you want to dive, keep your arms by your side or over your head, and kick, and when you want to come up, let your legs drag and paddle with your hands.'

We found a little basin among the rushes at the south end of the lake, about waist-deep and a rod or two wide, shaped like a sunfish's nest. Here we kicked and plashed for many a lesson, faithfully trying to imitate frogs; but the smooth, comfortable sliding gait of our amphibious teachers seemed hopelessly hard to learn. When we tried to kick frog-fashion, down went our heads as if weighted with lead the moment our feet left the ground.

One day it occurred to me to hold my breath as long as I could and let my head sink as far as it liked without paying any attention to it, and try to swim under the water instead of on the surface. This method was a great success, for at the very first trial I managed to cross the basin without touching bottom, and soon learned the use of my limbs. Then, of course swimming with my head above water soon became so easy that it seemed perfectly natural. David tried the plan with the same success. Then we began to count the number of times that we could swim around the basin without stopping to rest, and after twenty or thirty rounds failed to tire us, we proudly thought that a little more practice would make us as amphibious as frogs.

On the fourth of July of this swimming year one of the Lawson boys came to visit us, and we went down to spend the great warm day with the fishes and ducks and turtles. After gliding about on the smooth mirror water, telling stories and enjoying the company of the happy creatures about us, we rowed to our bathing-pool, and David and I went in to swim, while our companion fished from the boat a little out beyond the rushes. After a few turns in the pool, it occurred to me that it was now about time to try deep water. Swimming through the thick growth of rushes and lilies was somewhat dangerous, especially for a beginner, because one's arms and legs might be entangled among the long, limber stems; nevertheless I ventured and struck out boldly enough for the boat, where the water was twenty or thirty feet deep. When I reached the end of the little skiff I raised my right hand to take hold of it, to surprise Lawson, whose back was toward me and who was not aware of my approach; but I failed to reach high enough, and, of course, the weight of my arm and the stroke against the over-leaning stern of the boat shoved me down and I sank, struggling, frightened and confused. As soon as my feet touched the bottom, I slowly rose to the surface, but before I could get breath enough to call for help, sank back again and lost all control of myself. After sinking and rising I don't know how many times, some water got into my lungs and I began to drown. Then suddenly my mind seemed to clear. I remembered that I could swim underwater, and, making a desperate struggle toward the shore, I reached a point where, with my toes on the bottom, I got my mouth above the surface, gasped for help, and was pulled into the boat.

This humiliating accident spoiled the day, and we all agreed to keep it a profound secret. My sister Sarah had heard my cry for help and on our arrival at the house inquired what had happened. 'Were you drowning, John? I heard you cry you couldna get oot.' Lawson made haste to reply 'Oh, no! He was joist haverin.'

I was very much ashamed of myself, and at night, after calmly reviewing the affair, concluded that there had been no reasonable cause for the accident, and that I ought to punish myself for so nearly losing my life from unmanly fear. Accordingly at the very first opportunity I stole away to the lake by myself, got into my boat, and instead of going back to the old swimming-bowl for further practice, or to try to do sanely and well what I had so ignominiously failed to do in my first adventure, that is, to swim out through the rushes and lilies, I rowed directly out to the middle of the lake, stripped, stood up on the seat in the stern, and with grim deliberation took a header and dove straight down thirty or forty feet, turned easily, and, letting my feet drag, paddled straight to the surface with my hands as Father had at first directed me to do. I then swam round the boat, glorying in my suddenly acquired confidence and victory over myself, climbed into it, and dived again, with the same triumphant success. I think I went down four or five times, and each time as I made the dive-spring, shouted aloud, 'Take that!' feeling that was getting most gloriously even with myself.

Never again from that day to this have I lost control of myself in water. If suddenly thrown overboard at sea in the dark, or even while asleep, I think I would immediately right myself in a way some would call instinct, rise among the waves, catch my breath, and try to plan what would better be done. Never was victory over self more complete. I have been a good swimmer ever since. At a slow gait I think I could swim all day in smooth water moderate in temperature. When I was a student at Madison, I used to go on long swimming-journeys, called exploring expeditions, along the south shore of Lake Mendota, on Saturdays, sometimes alone, sometimes with another amphibious explorer by the name of Fuller.

~~~~~

BLACK FEMINIST POET AUDRE LORDE (1934–1992) was born in New York City to parents who were immigrants from Grenada. She was nearsighted to the point of being legally blind and grew up listening to West Indian songs and poems from her mother, which helped to inspire her love of the spoken word. Here, in a galvanising metaphor, Audre recalls her father teaching her to swim.

'Dropped into the inevitable'

A Question of Climate by Audre Lorde[10]

I learned to be honest
the way I learned to swim
dropped into the inevitable
my father's thumbs in my hairless armpits
about to give way
I am trying
to surface carefully
remembering
the water's shadow-legged musk
cannons of salt exploding
my nostrils' rage
and for years
my powerful breaststroke
was a declaration of war.

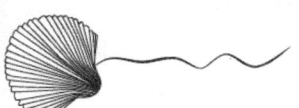

EUGENIE CLARK (1922–2015), AN AMERICAN marine biologist known as 'the shark lady', researched fish and shark behaviour. Her 1953 autobiography, *Lady With a Spear*, recalls her enjoyment of killing and eating tropical fish, something a scientist would be unlikely to do now. This, though, did not interfere with her admiration for sea creatures.

When the blockbuster film *Jaws* led to an increase in fear of sharks, Clark took the author of the book, Peter Benchley, on a dive to swim with sharks. 'When you see a shark underwater,' she said, 'you should say, "How lucky I am to see this beautiful animal in his environment."'

Eugenie's first swimming teacher was Yumico Motomi, her Japanese American mother, who was widowed when her daughter was two.

'We chewed gum and then plugged it into our ears before our first dip.'
The Lady and the Sharks by Eugenie Clark[11]

My mother began taking me to the beach before I was two years old. She had once been a swimming teacher and liked the water almost more than I did. My whole family—that is to say, grandma, uncle, and mama—all loved the beach. And all of them were expert swimmers. My uncle did fancy diving. I'd call my friends over to watch him and talk loudly so everyone could hear: 'There's my uncle. Watch him now, he's going to do a somersault.'

But it was with a quieter and secret pleasure that I watched my mother. Her strokes were rhythmical and graceful, and she swam long distances effortlessly. When she came out of the water she would take off her bathing-cap, and her jet-black hair, which she usually wore pinned up in conservative Japanese fashion, fell down to her hips. She looked more Oriental then than in the pictures I'd seen of her in kimonos when she was a young girl in Japan; she looked like a pearl-diver of the Orient. When I overheard the admiring remarks that strangers made about her, I didn't claim her as I did my uncle; I just listened quietly, secure in the knowledge that soon she would call me over and everyone would know she was my mother.

One of the first things that intrigued me about mama swimming was that she put chewing-gum in her ears. I didn't know why she did it, but it looked like a chic thing to do. So the first time I was allowed to chew gum, I lost no time stuffing it into my ears—along with much of my hair. But I soon learned the technique as well as the reason for it. Gum can be moulded to the exact shape of the ear opening, as a plug to keep the water out, and natural wax prevents it from sticking in the ear. I got a big kick out of the ritual of sitting on the beach with mama while we chewed gum and then plugged it into our ears before our first dip. It made me feel like a professional swimmer.

———~———

IN HIS EARLY LIFE, BENJAMIN Franklin's family owned slaves. But during his time in London and Paris, Franklin realised the inhumanity of this and he demanded that, when the United States became an independent country, it should abolish slavery. In 1787, at the age of eighty-one, Franklin became President of the Abolition Society and petitioned Congress on behalf of the society, requesting that they grant liberty 'to those unhappy men who alone in this land of freedom are degraded into perpetual bondage'.

In his memoirs, Franklin ascribed the adeptness in swimming he acquired as a child to studying *The Art of Swimming* by Thévenot. But, always an innovator, he was not content with the usual mode of getting along in the water. Here, in a letter to his friend Jacques Barbeu-Dubourg, Franklin recalls his unconventional approach.

'This singular mode of swimming.'
'Letters and Papers on Philosophical Subjects' in *The Works of Benjamin Franklin* by Jared Sparks (editor)[12]

When I was a boy I amused myself one day with flying a paper kite; and approaching the bank of a pond, which was near a mile broad, I tied the string to a stake, and the kite ascended to a very considerable height above the pond, while I was swimming. In a little time, being desirous of amusing myself with my kite, and enjoying at the same time the pleasure of swimming, I returned; and loosing from the stake the string with the little stick which was fastened to it, went again into the water, where I found, that, lying on my back and holding the stick in my hands, I was drawn along the surface of the water in a very agreeable manner.

Having then engaged another boy to carry my clothes round the pond, to a place which I pointed out to him on the other side, I began to cross the pond with my kite, which carried me quite over without the least fatigue, and with the greatest pleasure imaginable. I was only obliged occasionally to halt a little in my course, and resist its progress, when it appeared that, by following too quick, I lowered the kite too much; by doing which occasionally I made it rise again. I have never since that time practised this singular mode of swimming, though I think it not impossible to cross in this manner from Dover to Calais. The packet-boat, however, is still preferable.

CHAPTER III

The Right to Swim

EVEN WHEN SLAVERY WAS ENDED in the United States in 1865, almost a century after the American Revolution, the discrimination and oppression faced by Black people continued. So the experience of Black children, especially in the USA, was not the same as that of white children.

In the hot summer of 1919, a seventeen-year-old Black youth called Eugene Williams was playing on a raft that drifted into a beach area regarded as 'white' and was killed by rocks thrown at him. When the police refused to arrest the man who threw the rocks, it sparked a race riot.

Richard Wright, who became one of America's best-known Black authors, was eleven years old that summer and had a part-time job delivering the campaigning Black newspaper *The Chicago Defender*, so he would have been aware of this event — and others like it. In her paper *Dangerous Refuge, Richard Wright and the Swimming Hole*, Professor Melissa Ryan explores this and other incidents that inspired the short story, which appears in Wright's first published collection *Uncle Tom's Children*.

It is set in rural Mississippi, where the horsing around of a group of adolescent friends turns into a violent ordeal that leaves three out of four of them dead.

The boys decide to go swimming in a swimming hole where Blacks aren't allowed. After their bathe, they are lying sunning themselves when a white woman appears. The woman, who has been taught to fear Black males, is standing close to the pile of their clothes – and when they move towards her to retrieve them, she screams. A man appears with a gun and shoots two of the boys dead. In a struggle, another boy shoots him. The story ends with a third of the four boys being lynched, while the narrator escapes north to Chicago.

'LAS ONE INS A OL DEAD DOG!'
'Big Boy Leaves Home' by Richard Wright[13]

They came to the swimming hole . . .

Bobo pointed.

'See the sign over yonder?'

'Yeah.'

'Whut it say?'

'NO TRESPASSIN,' read Lester.

'Know whut tha mean?'

'Mean ain no dogs n niggers erllowed,' said Buck.

'Waal, wes here now,' said Big Boy. 'Ef he ketched us even like this thered be trouble, so we just as waal go on in . . .'

'Ahm wid the nex one!'

'Ahll go ef anybody else goes!'

Big Boy looked carefully in all directions. Seeing nobody, he began jerking off his overalls.

'LAS ONE INS A OL DEAD DOG!'

'THAS YO MA!'

'THAS YO PA!'

'THAS BOTH YO MA N YO PA!'

They jerked off their clothes and threw them in a pile under a tree. Thirty seconds later they stood, black and naked, on the edge of the hole under a sloping embankment. Gingerly Big Boy touched the water with his foot.

'Man, this waters col,' he said.

'Ahm gonna put mah cloes back on,' said Bobo, withdrawing his foot.

Big Boy grabbed him about the waist.

'Like hell yuh is!'

'Git outta the way, nigger!' Bobo yelled.

'Thow im in!' said Lester.

'Duck im!'

Bobo crouched, spread his legs, and braced himself against Big Boy's body. Locked in each other's arms, they tussled on the edge of the hole, neither able to throw the other.

'C'mon, les me n yuh push em in.'

'O.K.'

Laughing, Lester and Buck gave the two locked bodies a running push. Big Boy and Bobo splashed, sending up silver spray in the sunlight. When Big Boy's head came up he yelled:

'Yuh bastard!'

'The wuz yo ma yuh pushed!' said Bobo, shaking his head to clear the water from his eyes.

They did a surface dive, came up and struck out across the creek. The muddy water foamed. They swam back, waded into shallow water, breathing heavily and blinking eyes.

'C'mon in!'

'Man, the water's fine!'

Lester and Buck hesitated.

'Les wet em,' Big Boy whispered to Bobo.

Before Lester and Buck could back away, they were dripping wet from handfuls of scooped water.

'Hey, quit!'

'Gawddam, nigger; the waters col!'

'C'mon in!' called Big Boy

'We just as waal go on in now,' said Buck.

'Look n see ef anybody's comin.'

Kneeling, they squinted among the trees.

'Ain nobody.'

'C'mon, les go.'

They waded in slowly, pausing each few steps to catch their breath. A desperate water battle began. Closing eyes and backing away, they shunted water into one another's faces with the flat palms of hands.

'Hey, cut it out!'

'Yeah, Ahm bout drownin!'

They came together in water up to their navels, blowing and blinking. Big Boy ducked, upsetting Bobo.

'Look out, nigger!'

'Don holler so loud!'

'Yeah, they kin hear yo ol big mouth a mile erway.'

'This waters too col fer me.'

'Thas cause it rained yistiddy.'

They swam across and back again.

'Ah wish we hada bigger place t swim in.

'The white folks got plenty swimming pools n we ain got none.'

'Ah useta swim in the ol Missippi when we lived in Vicksburg.'

Big Boy put his head under the water and blew his breath. A sound came like that of a hippopotamus.

'C'mon, les be hippos.'

Each went to a corner of the creek and put his mouth dust below the surface and blew like a hippopotamus. Tiring, they came and sat under the embankment.

'Look like Ah gotta chill.'

'Me too.'

'Les stay here n dry off.'

'Jeeesus, Ahm col!'

They kept still in the sun, suppressing shivers. After some of the water had dried off their bodies they began to talk through clattering teeth.

'Whut would yuh do ef ol man Harveyd come erlong rlg t now?'

'Run like hells.'

'Man, Ahd run so fas hed thinka black streaka lightnin shot pass im.'

'But spose he hada gun?'

'Aw nigger, shut up!'

They were silent. They ran their hands over wet, trembling legs, brushing water away. Then their eyes watched the sun sparkling on the restless creek.

Far away a train whistled.

'There goes number seven!'

'Headin fer up Noth!'

'Blazin it down the line!'

'Lawd, Ahm goin Noth some day.'

'Me too, man.'

'They say coloured folks up Noth is got ekual rights.'

They grew pensive. A black-winged butterfly hovered at the water's edge. A bee droned. From somewhere came the sweet scent of honeysuckles. Dimly they could hear sparrows twittering in the woods. They rolled from side to side, letting sunshine dry their skins and warm their blood. They plucked blades of grass and chewed them.

'Oh!'

They looked up, their lips parting.

A white woman, poised on the edge of the opposite embankment, stood directly in front of them, her hat in her hand and her hair lit by the sun.

THE TITLE OF WRIGHT'S STORY refers to *Uncle Tom's Cabin* by Harriet Beecher Stowe, which was first published in 1852, more than a decade before slavery was abolished in America. Though not specifically intended for children, it was designed, as many books were in those days, to be read aloud in a family setting, with a dramatic, episodic structure. It was read across the world and for many white people it was an eye-opener to the violence and injustice of slavery. The book was a milestone in the Abolitionist campaign – when Abraham Lincoln met Stowe in 1862, he is supposed to have said: 'So you're the little woman who wrote the book that made this great war!'

Like much Victorian fiction, the lead characters are pattern-cards of moral rectitude. The audience would have understood the Christ allegory in the central figure of Tom, who refuses to escape when he is sold down the river (where conditions were worse), because of his Christian principles. Once aboard a steamboat and in the charge of brutal slave dealer Haley, Tom's situation improves after he dives into the Mississippi to rescue the young daughter of a wealthy passenger who has fallen overboard.

But the true horror of slavery is conveyed through the fate of the minor characters. Here, a young woman, Lucy, has been tricked into boarding the steamboat by her owner, who told her she is going to be reunited with her husband. Instead, she has been sold to Haley, who then sells her baby to a fellow traveller.

'He heard a splash in the water.'
Uncle Tom's Cabin by Harriet Beecher Stowe[14]

It was a bright, tranquil evening when the boat stopped at the wharf at Louisville. The woman had been sitting with her baby in her arms, now wrapped in a heavy sleep. When she heard the name of the place called out, she hastily laid the child down in a little cradle formed by the hollow among the boxes, first carefully spreading under it her cloak; and then she sprung to the side of the boat, in hopes that, among the various hotel-waiters who thronged the wharf, she might see her husband. In this hope, she pressed forward to the front rails, and, stretching far over them, strained her eyes intently on the moving heads on the shore, and the crowd pressed in between her and the child.

'Now's your time,' said Haley, taking the sleeping child up, and handing him to the stranger. 'Don't wake him up, and set him to crying, now; it would make a devil of a fuss with the gal.' The man took the bundle carefully, and was soon lost in the crowd that went up the wharf.

When the boat, creaking, and groaning, and puffing, had loosed from the wharf, and was beginning slowly to strain herself along, the woman returned to her old seat. The trader was sitting there,—the child was gone!

'Why, why,—where?' she began, in bewildered surprise.

'Lucy,' said the trader, 'your child's gone; you may as well know it first as last. You see, I know'd you couldn't take him down south; and

I got a chance to sell him to a first-rate family, that'll raise him better than you can.'

But the woman did not scream. The shot had passed too straight and direct through the heart, for cry or tear. Dizzily she sat down. Her slack hands fell lifeless by her side. Her eyes looked straight forward, but she saw nothing. All the noise and hum of the boat, the groaning of the machinery, mingled dreamily to her bewildered ear; and the poor, dumb-stricken heart had neither cry not tear to show for its utter misery. She was quite calm.

The trader, who, considering his advantages, was almost as humane as some of our politicians, seemed to feel called on to administer such consolation as the case admitted of.

'I know this yer comes kinder hard, at first, Lucy,' said he; 'but such a smart, sensible gal as you are, won't give way to it. You see it's *necessary*, and can't be helped!'

'O! don't, Mas'r, don't!' said the woman, with a voice like one that is smothering.

'You're a smart wench, Lucy,' he persisted; 'I mean to do well by ye, and get ye a nice place down river; and you'll soon get another hus-band,—such a likely gal as you—'

'O! Mas'r, if you *only* won't talk to me now,' said the woman, in a voice of such quick and living anguish that the trader felt that there was something at present in the case beyond his style of operation. He got up, and the woman turned away, and buried her head in her cloak.

The trader walked up and down for a time, and occasionally stopped and looked at her.

'Takes it hard, rather,' he soliloquised, 'but quiet, tho';—let her sweat a while; she'll come right, by and by!'

Night came on,—night calm, unmoved, and glorious, shining down

38

with her innumerable and solemn angel eyes, twinkling, beautiful, but silent. There was no speech nor language, no pitying voice or helping hand, from that distant sky. One after another, the voices of business or pleasure died away; all on the boat were sleeping, and the ripples at the prow were plainly heard. Tom stretched himself out on a box, and there, as he lay, he heard, ever and anon, a smothered sob or cry from the prostrate creature,—'O! what shall I do? O Lord! O good Lord, do help me!' and so, ever and anon, until the murmur died away in silence.

At midnight, Tom waked, with a sudden start. Something black passed quickly by him to the side of the boat, and he heard a splash in the water. No one else saw or heard anything. He raised his head,—the woman's place was vacant! He got up, and sought about him in vain. The poor bleeding heart was still, at last, and the river rippled and dimpled just as brightly as if it had not closed above it.

Patience! patience! ye whose hearts swell indignant at wrongs like these. Not one throb of anguish, not one tear of the oppressed, is forgotten by the Man of Sorrows, the Lord of Glory. In his patient, generous bosom he bears the anguish of a world. Bear thou, like him, in patience, and labor in love; for sure as he is God, 'the year of his redeemed *shall* come'.

The trader waked up bright and early, and came out to see to his live stock. It was now his turn to look about in perplexity.

'Where alive is that gal?' he said to Tom.

Tom, who had learned the wisdom of keeping counsel, did not feel called upon to state his observations and suspicions, but said he did not know.

'She surely couldn't have got off in the night at any of the landings, for I was awake, and on the lookout, whenever the boat stopped. I never trust these yer things to other folks.'

This speech was addressed to Tom quite confidentially, as if it was something that would be specially interesting to him. Tom made no answer. The trader searched the boat from stem to stern, among boxes, bales and barrels, around the machinery, by the chimneys, in vain.

'Now, I say, Tom, be fair about this yer,' he said, when, after a fruitless search, he came where Tom was standing. 'You know something about it, now. Don't tell me,—I know you do. I saw the gal stretched out here about ten o'clock, and ag'in at twelve, and ag'in between one and two; and then at four she was gone, and you was a sleeping right there all the time. Now, you know something,—you can't help it.'

'Well, Mas'r,' said Tom, 'towards morning something brushed by me, and I kinder half woke; and then I hearn a great splash, and then I clare woke up, and the gal was gone. That's all I know on 't.'

The trader was not shocked nor amazed; because, as we said before, he was used to a great many things that you are not used to. Even the awful presence of Death struck no solemn chill upon him. He had seen Death many times,—met him in the way of trade, and got acquainted with him,—and he only thought of him as a hard customer, that embarrassed his property operations very unfairly; and so he only swore that the gal was a baggage, and that he was devilish unlucky, and that, if things went on in this way, he should not make a cent on the trip. In short, he seemed to consider himself an ill-used man, decidedly; but there was no help for it, as the woman had escaped into a state which *never will* give up a fugitive,—not even at the demand of the whole glorious Union.

THE AMERICAN CLASSIC *Huckleberry Finn* has been brought to new audiences in Percival Everett's bestselling retelling *James*. Everett retains the main planks of the tale, in which teenage runaway Huck and escaped slave Jim make their way down the Mississippi river with many spills and encounters. In his satirical modern retelling, Everett has Jim adopt a 'slave' persona while in the presence of white people.

Mark Twain's original was published in 1885, after slavery had been abolished but while it was in living memory, and in a United States still riven by racist laws. Here is Twain's lyrical description of Huck and Jim's journey on the river and their swimming together.

'We slid into the river and had a swim.'
Huckleberry Finn by Mark Twain[15]

Two or three days and nights went by; I reckon I might say they swum by, they slid along so quiet and smooth and lovely. Here is the way we put in the time. It was a monstrous big river down there sometimes a mile and a half wide; we run nights, and laid up and hid daytime; soon as night was most gone we stopped navigating and tied up nearly always in the dead water under a towhead; and then cut young cottonwoods and willows, and hid the raft with them. Then we set out the lines.

Next we slid into the river and had a swim, so as to freshen up and cool off; then we set down on the sandy bottom where the water was about knee-deep, and watched the daylight come. Not a sound anywhere perfectly still just like the whole world was asleep, only sometimes the bullfrogs a-cluttering, maybe.

The first thing to see, looking away over the water, was a kind of dull line – that was the woods on t'other side; you couldn't make nothing else out; then a pale place in the sky; then more paleness spreading around; then the river softened up away off, and warn't black any more, but gray; you could see little dark spots drifting along ever so far away trading – scows, and such things; and long black streaks-rafts;

sometimes you could hear a sweep screaking; or jumbled-up voices, it was so still, and sounds come so far; and by and by you could see a streak on the water which you know by the look of the streak that there's a snag there in a swift current which breaks on it and makes that streak look that way; and you see the mist curl up off of the water, and the east reddens up, and the river, and you make out a log cabin in the edge of the woods, away on the bank on t'other side of the river, being a wood-yard, likely, and piled by them cheats so you can throw a dog through it anywhere; then the nice breeze springs up, and comes fanning you from over there, so cool and fresh and sweet to smell on account of the woods and the flowers; but sometimes not that way, because they've left dead fish laying around, gars and such, and they do get pretty rank; and next you've got the full day, and everything smiling in the sun, and the song-birds just going it!

A little smoke couldn't be noticed now, so we would take some fish off of the lines and cook up a hot breakfast. And afterwards we would watch the lonesomeness of the river, and kind of lazy along, and by and by lazy off to sleep. Wake up by and by, and look to see what done it, and maybe see a steamboat coughing along upstream, so far off towards the other side you couldn't tell nothing about her only whether she was a stern-wheel or side-wheel; then for about an hour there wouldn't be nothing to hear nor nothing to see – just solid lonesomeness. Next you'd see a raft sliding by, away off yonder, and maybe a galoot on it chopping, because they're most always doing it on a raft; you'd see the ax flash and come down – you don't hear nothing; you see that ax go up again, and by the time it's above the man's head then you hear the k'chunk! it had took all that time to come over the water.

CHAPTER IV

Parents on the Edge

SOMETIMES IT IS BY THE seashore that families have time to be together and let their relationships unfold. We start this section with an excerpt from a short story by one of the twentieth century's most subtle masters of the form, Andre Dubus – in which Peter struggles to connect with his children after divorce. He can't recreate the easy communication that he had when they lived together and, through the winter, their weekends involve trips by car to places of entertainment. When the summer comes at last, the beach becomes their sanctuary.

'He would always test the current first.'
'The Winter Father' by Andre Dubus[16]

Frenetic as they were he preferred weekends to the Wednesday nights when they ate together. At first, he thought it was shyness. Yet they talked easily, often about their work, theirs at school, his as a disc jockey. When he was not with the children, he spent much time thinking about what they said to each other. And he saw that, in his eight years as a father, he had been attentive, respectful, amusing; he had taught and disciplined. But no: not now; when they were too loud in the car or they fought, he held onto his anger, his heart buffeted with it, and spoke calmly as though to another man's children, for he was afraid that if he scolded as he had before, the day would be spoiled, they would not have the evening at home, the sleeping in the same house, to heal them, and they might not want to go with him next day or two nights from now or two days.

Peter acquires a girlfriend called Mary Ann.

She wanted a lover, she said, not love, not what it still did to men and women. He did not tell her he thought they were using each other in a way that might have been cynical, if it were not so frightening. He simply followed her, became one of those who make love with their friends. But she was his only woman friend, and he did not know how many men shared her. When she told him she would not be home this night or that weekend, he held his questions. He held onto his heart too, and forced himself to make her a part of the times when he was alone. He had married young, and life to him was surrounded by the sounds and touches of a family. Now in this foreign land he felt so vulnerably strange that at times it seemed near madness as he gave Mary Ann a function in his time, ranking somewhere among his running and his work. When the children asked about her, he said they were still friends . . .

He and the children went out every Sunday. And that was how the cold months passed, beginning with the New Year, because Peter and Norma had waited until after Christmas to end the marriage: the movies and sledding, museums and aquarium, the restaurants; always they were on the road, and whenever he looked at his car he thought of the children. How many conversations while looking through the windshield? How many times had the doors slammed shut and they re-entered or left his life? Winter ended slowly. April was cold and in May Peter and the children still wore sweaters or windbreakers, and on two weekends there was rain, and everything they did together was indoors. But when the month ended, Peter thought it was not the weather but the patterns of winter that had kept them driving from place to place.

Then it was June and they were out of school and Peter took his vacation. Norma worked, and by nine in the morning he and Kathi and David were driving to the sea. They took a large blanket and tucked its corners into the sand so it wouldn't flap in the wind, and they lay oiled in the sun. On the first day they talked of winter how they could feel the sun warming their ribs, as they had watched it warming the earth during the long thaw. It was a beach with gentle currents and a gradual slope out to sea but Peter told them, as he had every summer, about undertow: that if ever they were caught in one, they must not swim against it; they must let it take them out and then they must swim parallel to the beach until the current shifted and they could swim back in with it. He could not imagine his children being calm enough to do that, for he was afraid of water and only enjoyed body-surfing near the beach, but he told them anyway. Then he said it would not happen because he would always test the current first.

In those first two weeks the three of them ran into the water and body-surfed for only a few minutes, for it was too cold still, and they had to leave it until their flesh was warm again. They would not be able to stay in long until July. Peter showed them the different colours of summer, told them why on humid days the sky and ocean were paler blue, and on dry days they were darker, more beautiful and the trees they passed on the roads to the beach were brighter green. He bought a whiffle ball and bat and kept them in the trunk of his car and they played at the beach. The children dug holes, made castles, Peter watched, slept, and in late morning he ran.

From a large thermos they drank lemonade or juice; and they ate lunch all day, the children grazing on fruit and the sandwiches he had made before his breakfast. Then he took them to his apartment for showers, and they helped carry in the ice chest and thermos and blanket and their knapsack of clothes. Kathi and David still took turns showering first, and they stayed in longer, but now in summer the water was still hot when his turn came. Then he drove them home to Norma, his skin red and pleasantly burning; then tan.

When his vacation ended they spent all sunny weekends at the sea, and even grey days that were warm. The children became braver about the cold, and forced him to go in with them and body-surf. But they could stay longer than he could, and he left to lie on the blanket and watch them, to make sure they stayed in shallow water. He made them promise to wait on the beach while he ran. He went in the water to cool his body from the sun, but mostly he lay on the blanket, reading, and watching the children wading out to the breakers and riding them in. Kathi and David did not always stay together. One left to walk the beach alone. Another played with strangers, or children who were there most days too. One built a castle. Another body-surfed. And, often, one would come to the blanket and drink and take a sandwich from the ice chest, would sit eating and drinking beside Peter, offer him a bite, a swallow. And on all those beach days Peter's shyness and apprehension were gone.

It's the sea, he said to Mary Ann one night.

And it was: for on that day, a long Saturday at the beach, when he had all day felt peace and father-love and sun and salt water, he had understood why now in summer he and his children were as he had yearned for them to be in winter: they were no longer confined to car or buildings to remind them why they were there. The long beach and the sea were their lawn; the blanket their home; the ice chest and thermos their kitchen.

They lived as a family again. While he ran and David dug in the sand until he reached water and Kathi looked for pretty shells for her room, the blanket waited for them. It was the place they wandered back to: for food, for drink, for rest, their talk as casual as between children and father arriving, through separate doors, at the kitchen sink for water, the refrigerator for an orange. Then one left for the surf; another slept in the sun, lips stained with grape juice. He had wanted to tell the children about it, but it was too much to tell, and the beach was no place for such talk anyway, and he also guessed they knew.

So that afternoon when they were all lying on the blanket, on their backs, the children flanking him, he simply said: 'Divorced kids go to the beach more than married ones.'

'Why?' Kathi said.

'Because married people do chores and errands on weekends. No kid-days.'

'I love the beach,' David said.

'So do I,' Peter said.

He looked at Kathi.

'You don't like it, huh?'

She took her arm from her eyes and looked at him. His urge was to turn away. She looked at him for a long time; her eyes were too tender, too wise, and he wished she could have learned both later, and differently; in her eyes he saw the car in winter, heard its doors opening and closing, their talk and the sounds of heater and engine and tires on the road, and the places the car took them. Then she held his hand, and closed her eyes.

'I wish it was summer all year round,' she said.

~

ANNA KARENINA'S SISTER-IN-LAW, DOLLY, is a major character in Leo Tolstoy's complex, romantic masterpiece. Anna is unfaithful to her husband and, as a result, loses everything, including access to her son. Dolly's husband is unfaithful to her, too – but the outcome is very different. The couple drift apart and Dolly focuses her love on her children.

Here Dolly has retreated from her unhappy marriage and life in Moscow to spend summer in the countryside, with her children. They go swimming in the river after returning from church after taking Holy Communion (a rare event).

'To see the breathless faces of all her splashing cherubs was a great pleasure.'

Anna Karenina by Leo Tolstoy[17]

On the way home the children felt that something solemn had happened, and were very sedate. Everything went happily at home too; but at lunch Grisha began whistling, and, what was worse, was disobedient to the English governess, and was forbidden to have any tart. Darya Alexandrovna would not have let things go so far on such a day had she been present; but she had to support the English governess's authority, and she upheld her decision that Grisha should have no tart. This rather spoiled the general good humor. Grisha cried, declaring that Nikolinka had whistled too, and he was not punished, and that he wasn't crying for the tart—he didn't care—but at being unjustly treated. This was really too tragic, and Darya Alexandrovna made up her mind to persuade the English governess to forgive Grisha, and she went to speak to her. But on the way, as she passed the drawing-room, she beheld a scene, filling her heart with such pleasure that the tears came into her eyes, and she forgave the delinquent herself.

The culprit was sitting at the window in the corner of the drawing-room; beside him was standing Tanya with a plate. On the pretext of wanting to give some dinner to her dolls, she had asked the governess's permission to take her share of tart to the nursery, and had taken it instead to her brother. While still weeping over the injustice of his punishment, he was eating the tart, and kept saying through his sobs, 'Eat yourself; let's eat it together . . . together.'

On catching sight of their mother they were dismayed, but, looking into her face, they saw they were not doing wrong. They burst out laughing, and, with their mouths full of tart, they began wiping their smiling lips with their hands, and smearing their radiant faces all over with tears and jam.

'Mercy! Your new white frock! Tanya! Grisha!' said their mother, trying to save the frock, but with tears in her eyes, smiling a blissful, rapturous smile.

The new frocks were taken off, and orders were given for the little girls to have their blouses put on, and the boys their old jackets, and the wagonette to be harnessed; with Brownie, to the bailiff's annoyance, again in the shafts, to drive out for mushroom picking and bathing. A roar of delighted shrieks arose in the nursery, and never ceased till they had set off for the bathing-place.

They reached the river, put the horses under the birch trees, and went to the bathing-place. The coachman, Terenty, fastened the horses, who kept whisking away the flies, to a tree, and, treading down the grass, lay down in the shade of a birch and smoked his shag, while the never-ceasing shrieks of delight of the children floated across to him from the bathing-place.

Though it was hard work to look after all the children and restrain their wild pranks, though it was difficult too to keep in one's head and not mix up all the stockings, little breeches, and shoes for the different legs, and to undo and to do up again all the tapes and buttons, Darya Alexandrovna, who had always liked bathing herself, and believed it to be very good for the children, enjoyed nothing so much as bathing with all the children. To go over all those fat little legs, pulling on their stockings, to take in her arms and dip those little naked bodies, and to hear their screams of delight and alarm, to see the breathless faces with wide-open, scared, and happy eyes of all her splashing cherubs, was a great pleasure to her.

When half the children had been dressed, some peasant women in holiday dress, out picking herbs, came up to the bathing-shed and stopped shyly. Marya Philimonovna called one of them and handed her a sheet and a shirt that had dropped into the water for her to dry them, and Darya Alexandrovna began to talk to the women. At first they laughed behind their hands and did not understand her questions, but soon they grew bolder and began to talk, winning Darya Alexandrovna's heart at once by the genuine admiration of the children that they showed.

'My, what a beauty! as white as sugar,' said one, admiring Tanitchka, and shaking her head; 'but thin . . .'

'Yes, she has been ill.'

'And so they've been bathing you too,' said another to the baby.

'No; he's only three months old,' answered Darya Alexandrovna with pride.

'You don't say so!'

'And have you any children?'

'I've had four; I've two living—a boy and a girl. I weaned her last carnival.'

'How old is she?'

'Why, two years old.'

'Why did you nurse her so long?'

'It's our custom; for three fasts . . .'

And the conversation became most interesting to Darya Alexandrovna. What sort of time did she have? What was the matter with the boy? Where was her husband? Did it often happen?

Darya Alexandrovna felt disinclined to leave the peasant women, so interesting to her was their conversation, so completely identical were all their interests. What pleased her most of all was that she saw clearly what all the women admired more than anything was her having so many children, and such fine ones. The peasant women even made Darya Alexandrovna laugh, and offended the English governess, because she was the cause of the laughter she did not understand. One of the younger women kept staring at the Englishwoman, who was dressing after all the rest, and when she put on her third petticoat she could not refrain from the remark, 'My, she keeps putting on and putting on, and she'll never have done!' she said, and they all went off into roars.

IN HIS MEMOIR, *Letter to My Father*, Franz Kafka, who died in 1924 aged forty, remembers how he compared himself unfavourably to his father. Kafka always believed himself to be physically unattractive and too skinny – as an adult he was almost six foot tall and weighed just over eight stone (52 kilograms). Modern tastes, perhaps, are different and in recent years photos of his soulful face have been admiringly shared millions of times on TikTok with the hashtag #kafka.

'You were for me the measure of all things.'

Letter to My Father by Franz Kafka[18]

I remember, for instance, how we often undressed in the same bathing hut. There was I, skinny, weakly, slight; you strong, tall, broad. Even inside the hut I felt a miserable specimen, and what's more, not only in your eyes but in the eyes of the whole world, for you were for me the measure of all things. But then when we stepped out of the bathing hut before the people, you holding me by my hand, a little skeleton, unsteady, barefoot on the boards, frightened of the water, incapable of copying your swimming strokes, which you, with the best of intentions, but actually to my profound humiliation, kept on demonstrating, then I was frantic with desperation and at such moments all my bad experiences in all areas, fitted magnificently together. I felt best when you sometimes undressed first and I was able to stay behind in the hut alone and put off the disgrace of showing myself in public until at last you came to see what I was doing and drove me out of the hut. I was grateful to you for not seeming to notice my anguish, and besides, I was proud of my father's body.

~

V. S. NAIPAUL BASED THE journalist Mohun Biswas in *A House for Mr Biswas*, on his own father, and the son, Anand, on himself. The book, set in Trinidad, is considered the Nobel Prize winner's masterpiece. Here Mr Biswas goes swimming with two brothers-in-law he feels look down on him, and Anand. The dockland area has been partially dredged and the boy, who can't really swim, falls into a deep area and has to be hauled out.

'I opened my mouth to cry for help. Water filled it.'

A House for Mr Biswas by V. S. Naipaul[19]

After breakfast all the men – and this included Anand – went for a bathe at the harbour extension at Docksite. The sun was not out and the high, stationary clouds were touched with red. Ships were blurred in the distance; the level sea was like dark glass. Anand was left at the edge of the water, near the wall, and the men went ahead, their voices and splashings carrying far in the stillness. All at once the sun came out, the water blazed, and sounds were subdued.

Aware of his unimpressive physique, Mr Biswas began to clown; and, as he did more and more now, he tried to extend his clowning to Anand.

'Duck, boy!' he called. 'Duck and let us see how long you can stay under water.'

'No!' Anand shouted back. His abrupt denial of his father's authority had become part of the clowning.

'You hear the boy?' Mr Biswas said to Owad and Shekhar. He spoke an obscene Hindi epigram which had always amused them and which they now associated with him.

'You know what I feel like doing?' he said a little later. 'See that rowing boat there, by the wall? Let us untie it. By tomorrow morning it will be in Venezuela.'

'And let us throw you in it,' Shekhar said.

They chased Mr Biswas, caught him, held him above the water while he laughed and squirmed, his calves swinging like hammocks. One, they counted, swinging him. Two – Suddenly he became affronted and angry.

'Three!' The smooth water slapped his belly and chest and forehead like something hard and hot. Surfacing, his back to them, he took some time to rearrange his hair, in reality wiping away the tears that had come to his eyes. The pause was long enough to tell Owad and Shekhar that he was angry. They were embarrassed: and he was recognizing the unreasonableness of his anger when Shekhar said, 'Where is Anand?'

Mr Biswas didn't turn. 'The boy is all right. Ducking. His grandfather was a champion diver.'

Owad laughed.

'Ducking, hell!' Shekhar said, and began swimming towards the wall.

There was no sign of Anand. In the shadow of the wall the rowing boat barely rocked above its reflection. Silently Mr Biswas and Owad watched Shekhar. He dived. Mr Biswas scooped up a handful of water and let it fall on his head. Some of it ran down his face; some of it sprinkled the sea. Shekhar reappeared near the sea-wall, shook the water from his head and dived again. Mr Biswas began to wade towards the wall. Owad began to swim. Mr Biswas began to swim.

Shekhar surfaced again, near the rowingboat. There was alarm on his face. He was holding Anand under his left arm and was pulling strongly with his right. Owad and Mr Biswas moved towards him. He shouted to them to keep away. All at once he stopped pulling with his right hand, stood up, and was only waist-high in water. Behind him, in shadow, the rowing boat barely moved.

They carried Anand to the top of the wall and rolled him. Then Shekhar did some kneading exercises on his thin back. Mr Biswas stood by, noticing only the large safety pin – one of Shamna's, doubtless – on Anand's blue striped shirt, which lay in the small heap of his clothes. Anand spluttered. His expression was one of anger. He said, 'I was walking to the boat.'

'I told you to stay where you were,' Mr Biswas said, angry too.

'And the bottom of the sea drop away.'

'The dredging,' Shekhar said. He had not lost his look of alarm.

'The sea just drop away' Anand cried, lying on his back, covering his face with a crooked arm. He spoke as one insulted.

Owad said, 'Anyway, you've got the record for ducking, Shompo.'

'Shut up!' Anand screamed. He began to cry, rubbing his legs on the hard, cracked ground, then turning over on his belly. Mr Biswas took up the shirt with the safety pin and handed it to Anand. Anand snatched the shirt and said, 'Leave me.'

'We shoulda leave you,' Mr Biswas said, when you was there, ducking.' As soon as he spoke the last word he regretted it.

'Yes!' Anand screamed. You shoulda leave me.' He got up and, going to his heap of clothes, began to dress furiously, forcing his clothes over his wet and gritty skin. I am never going to come out with any of you again.' His eyes were small and red, the lids swollen.

He walked away from them, quickly, his small body silhouetted against the sun, across the weed-ridden mud flat. Unused, his towel remained rolled, a large bundle below his arm . . .

The next day Mr Biswas wrote an angry article about the lack of warning notices at Docksite. In the afternoon Anand came home from school a little more composed and, extraordinarily, without being asked, took out a copy book from his bag and handed it to Mr Biswas, who was in the hammock in the back verandah. Then Anand went to change.

The copy book contained Anand's English compositions, which reflected the vocabulary and ideals of Anand's teacher as well as Anand's obsession with the stylistic device of the noun followed by a dash, an adjective and the noun again: for example, 'the robbers – the ruthless robbers'.

The last composition was headed 'A Day by the Seaside'. Below that the phrases supplied by the teacher had been copied down: project a visit – feverish preparations – eager anticipation – laden hampers – wind blowing through open car – spirits overflowing into song – graceful curve of coconut trees – arc of golden sand – crystalline water – pounding surf – majestic rollers – energetically battling the waves – cries of delirious joy – grateful shade of coconut trees – glorious sunset – sad to leave – memory to be cherished in future days – looking forward in eager anticipation to paying a return visit.

Mr Biswas was familiar with the clarity and optimism of the teacher's vision, and he expected Anand to write: With anticipation – eager anticipation – we projected a visit to the seaside and we made preparations – feverish preparations – and then on the appointed morning we struggled with hampers – laden hampers – into the motorcar. For in these compositions Anand and his fellows knew nothing but luxury.

But in this last composition there were no dashes and repetitions; no hampers, no motorcar, no golden arcs of sand; only a walk to Docksite, a concrete sea-wall and liners in the distance. Mr Biswas read on, anxious to share the pain of the previous day. 'I raised my hand but I did not know if it got to the top. I opened my mouth to cry for help. Water filled it. I thought I was going to die and I closed my eyes because I did not want to look at the water.': The composition ended with a denunciation of the sea. None of the teacher's phrases had been used but the composition had been given twelve marks out of ten. Anand had come back to the verandah and was having his tea at the table. Mr Biswas wished to be close to him. He would have done anything to make up for the solitude of the previous day. He said, 'Come and sit down here and go through the composition with me.'

Anand became impatient. He was pleased by the marks but was fed up with the composition and even a little ashamed of it. He had been made to read it out to the class, and the confession that he had not struggled with laden hampers into a car and driven to palm-fringed beaches but had walked to common Docksite had caused some laughter. So had the sentences: 'I opened my mouth to cry for help. Water filled it.'

'Come,' Mr Biswas said, making room in the hammock.

'No!' Anand shouted. But there was no one to laugh.

Mr Biswas's hurt turned to anger. Go and cut me a whip, he said, getting out of the hammock. 'Go on. Quick, sharp.'

CHAPTER V

Adventure

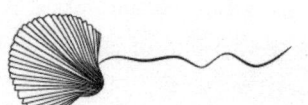

THERE ARE THOUSANDS OF ADVENTURE stories for children and adults in which people are shipwrecked, hide from pursuers by lurking underwater while breathing through reeds, or battle underwater monsters. *The Weirdstone of Brisingamen* by Alan Garner, *The Island of Adventure* by Enid Blyton and *The Beach* by Alex Garland all have scenes where the protagonists have to hold their breath and swim out through flooded tunnels. Terrifying. As a child, I loved a series of books about some children who found a secret cave behind a waterfall in the Hebrides that they entered by diving through a pool, but I have never been able to find these again. Here is a selection of dramatic scenes.

In the novel by John Irving published in 1989, Owen Meany is a child of very short stature, the best friend of the narrator. It's a darkly comic narrative set against the backdrop of the Vietnam War. Here Meany and his schoolfriends go swimming in the dangerously deep gravel quarry that his father owns.

'WHAT WERE YOU WAITING FOR? BUBBLES?'
A Prayer for Owen Meany by John Irving[20]

And for all the dirty tricks we played on him, he tricked us only once. We were allowed to swim in one of his father's quarries only if we entered and left the water one at a time and with a stout rope tied around our waists. One did not actually swim in those quarry lakes, which were rumoured to be as deep as the ocean, they were as cold as the ocean, even in late summer: they were as black and still as pools of oil. it was not the cold that made you want to rush out as soon as you'd jumped in; it was the unmeasured depth – our fear of what was on the bottom, and how far below us the bottom was. Owen's father, Mr Meany, insisted on the rope – insisted on one-at-at-em in-and-out. It was one of the few parental rules from my childhood that remained unbroken, except once – by Owen. It was never a rule that any of us cared to challenge; no one wanted to untie the rope and plunge without hope of rescue toward the unknown bottom.

But one fine August day, Owen Meany untied the rope, underwater, and he swam underwater to some hidden crevice on the rocky shore while we waited for him to rise. When he didn't surface, we pulled up the rope and waited for him to rise. Because we believed that Owen was nearly weightless, we refused to believe what our arms told us – that he was not at the end of the rope. We didn't believe he was gone until we had the bulging knot at the rope's end out of the water. What a silence that was! – interrupted only by the drops of water from the rope falling into the quarry.

No one called his name; no one dove in to look for him. In that water, no one could see! I prefer to believe that we would have gone in to look for him – if he'd given us just a few more seconds to gather up our nerve – but Owen decided that our response was altogether too slow and uncaring. He swam out from the crevice at the opposite shore; he moved as lightly as a water bug across the terrifying hole that reached, we were sure, to the bottom of the earth. He swam to us, angrier than we'd ever seen him.

'TALK ABOUT HURTING SOMEONE'S FEELINGS!' he cried

'WHAT WERE YOU WAITING FOR? BUBBLES? DO YOU THINK I'M A FISH? WASN'T ANYONE GOING TO TRY TO FIND ME?'

'You scared us, Owen,' one of us said. We were too scared to defend ourselves, if there was any defending ourselves – ever – in regard to Owen.

'YOU LET ME DROWN!' Owen said. 'YOU DIDN'T DO ANYTHING! YOU JUST WATCHED ME DROWN! I'M ALREADY DEAD!' he told us. 'REMEMBER THAT: YOU LET ME DIE.'

～～～

JOHN BUCHAN IS REMEMBERED PRINCIPALLY for *The Thirty-Nine Steps*, which, even Buchan admitted, Alfred Hitchcock improved when he turned it into a movie. But apart from that, Buchan's best is a classic of the adventure genre, beloved of youths and adults alike. In *John Macnab*, published in the 1920s, three eminent middle-aged men have lost their spark and are suffering from ennui. One of them consults a doctor who gives him this famous yet unorthodox advice.

The doctor was smiling. "If you ask my professional advice," he said, "I am bound to tell you that medical science has no suggestion to offer. If you consult me as a friend, I advise you to steal a horse in some part of the world where a horse thief is usually hanged."

The trio create a persona called John Macnab and challenge three Scottish landowners to stop them from poaching game – risking scandal if they are caught. Even today in certain circles 'a Macnab' means bagging a stag, a salmon and a brace of grouse in a day. (A Royal Macnab adds the challenge of bedding a lady.)

In this extract, Lamancha and the gamekeeper Wattie are poaching a stag from the estate of a wealthy industrialist, in the course of which they do something like what we would now call gorge-walking.

'It was a job for a merman rather than for breeched human beings.'
John Macnab by John Buchan[21]

At first sight the place seemed to be without deer. Lamancha, scanning it with his glass, could detect no living thing among the debris. Wattie was calling fiercely on his Maker. "God, it's the auld hero," he muttered, his eyes glued to his telescope. At last Lamancha got his glasses adjusted, and saw what his companion saw. Far up the corrie, on a patch of herbage – the last before the desert of the rocks began – stood three stags. Two were ordinary beasts, shootable, for they must have weighed sixteen or seventeen stone, but with inconsiderable heads. The third was no heavier, but he had a head like a blasted pine going back fast, for the beast was old, but still with thirteen clearly marked points and a most noble spread of horn.

A long circuit was necessary, happily in good cover, and the stream was not rejoined till at a point where its channel bore to the south, so that their wind would not be carried to the beasts below the knoll. After that it seemed advisable to Wattie to keep to the water, which was flowing in a deep-cut bed. It was a job for a merman rather than for breeched human beings, for Wattie would permit of no rising to a horizontal or even to a kneeling position.

The burn entered at their collars and flowed steadily through their shirts to an exit at their knees. Never had men been so comprehensively and continuously wet. Lamancha's right arm ached with pulling the rifle along the bank – he always insisted on carrying his weapon himself – while his body was submerged in the icy outflow of Sgurr Dearg's springs. The pressure of Wattie's foot in his face halted him. Blinking through the spray, he saw his leader's head raised stiffly to the alert in the direction of a little knoll. Even in the thick weather he could detect a pair of bat-like ears, and he realised that these ears were twitching. It did not need Wattie's whisper of "the auld bitch" to reveal the enemy. The two lay in the current for what seemed to Lamancha at least half an hour. He had enough hill craft to recognise that their one hope was to stick to the channel, for only thus was there a chance of their presence being unrevealed by the wind. But the channel led them very close to the hind. If the brute chose to turn her foolish head they would be within view.

With desperate slowness, an inch at a time, Wattie moved upwards. He signed to Lamancha to wait while he traversed a pool where only his cap and nose showed above the water. Then came a peat wallow, when his face seemed to be ground into the moss, and his limbs to be splayed like a frog's and to move with frog-like jerks. After that was a little cascade, and, beyond, the shelter of a big boulder which would get him out of the hind's orbit. Lamancha watched this strange progress with one eye; the other was on the twitching ears. Mercifully all went well, and Wattie's stern disappeared round a corner of rock. He laboured to follow with the same precision. The pool was easy enough except for the trailing of the rifle. The peat was straightforward going, though in his desire to follow his leader's example he dipped his face so deep in the black slime that his nostrils were plugged with it, and some got into his eyes which he dared not try to remove. But the waterfall was a snag. It was no light task to draw himself up against the weight of descending water, and at the top he lay panting for a second, damming up the flow with his body. Then he moved on; but the mischief had been done. For the sound of the release of the pent-up stream had struck a foreign note on the hind's ear. It was an unfamiliar noise among the many familiar ones which at the moment filled the corrie. She turned her head sharply, and saw something in the burn which she did not quite understand. Lamancha, aware of her scrutiny, lay choking, with the water running into his nose; but the alarm had been given. The hind turned her head, and trotted off up-wind. The next he knew was Wattie at his elbow making wild signals to him to rise and follow. Cramped and staggering, he lumbered after him away from the stream into a moraine of great granite blocks.

"We're no twa hundred yards from the stags," the guide whispered. "The auld bitch will move them, but please God we'll get a shot."

LAURA INGALLS WILDER'S *Little House on the Prairie* has sold 60 million copies since its first publication in 1935. Laura's account of her by-then distant childhood (she was born in 1867) is written from the point of view of an immigrant family crossing the American continent by wagon and then struggling to farm on the prairie.

The narrative has been criticised for lack of awareness of the perspective of Indigenous people. Ma is distrustful of them, Pa negotiates with a local chief, while big-eyed Laura simply observes. It is important to be aware of the book's point of view, and the way nostalgia colours Wilder's remembrance of the past. But her stories of this intrepid family dealing as a team with whatever nature throws at them are inspiring. I think 'Pa' is one of the most lovable fathers in children's fiction; warm, resourceful, affectionate and, at moments of leisure, always ready to take out his fiddle and play some Irish jigs.

When reading this passage to my children when they were young, I would point out that the children obey Ma's instructions without question in an emergency, and ask how we would fare in a similar situation.

'Then Pa's voice frightened Laura. It said, "Take them, Caroline!"'

Little House on the Prairie by Laura Ingalls Wilder[22]

'This creek's pretty high,' Pa said. 'But I guess we can make it all right. You can see this is a ford, by the old wheel ruts. What do you say, Caroline?'

'Whatever you say, Charles,' Ma answered.

Pet and Patty lifted their wet noses. They pricked their ears forward, looking at the creek; then they pricked them backward to hear what Pa would say. They sighed and laid their soft noses together to whisper to each other.

'I'll tie down the wagon-cover,' Pa said. He climbed down from the seat, unrolled the canvas sides and tied them firmly to the wagon box. Then he pulled the rope at the back, so that the canvas puckered together in the middle, leaving only a tiny round hole, too small to see through.

Mary huddled down on the bed. She did not like fords; she was afraid of the rushing water. But Laura was excited; she liked the splashing.

The wagon went forward softly in mud. Water began to splash against the wheels. The splashing grew louder. The wagon shook as the noisy water struck at it. Then all at once the wagon lifted and balanced and swayed. It was a lovely feeling. The noise stopped, and Ma said, sharply,

'Lie down, girls!'

Quick as a flash, Mary and Laura dropped flat on the bed. When

Ma spoke like that, they did as they were told. Ma's arm pulled a smothering blanket over them, heads and all.

'Be still, just as you are. Don't move!' she said.

Mary did not move; she was trembling and still. But Laura could not help wriggling a little bit. She did so want to see what was happening. She could feel the wagon swaying and turning; the splashing was noisy again, and again it died away. Then Pa's voice frightened Laura. It said, 'Take them, Caroline!' The wagon lurched; there was a sudden heavy splash beside it. Laura sat straight up and clawed the blanket from her head.

Pa was gone. Ma sat alone, holding tight to the reins with both hands. Mary hid her face in the blanket again, but Laura rose up farther. She couldn't see the creek bank. She couldn't see anything in front of the wagon but water rushing at it. And in the water, three heads; Pet's head and Patty's head and Pa's small, wet head. Pa's fist in the water was holding tight to Pet's bridle.

Laura could faintly hear Pa's voice through the rushing of the water. It sounded calm and cheerful, but she couldn't hear what he said. He was talking to the horses. Ma's face was white and scared. 'Lie down, Laura,' Ma said.

Laura lay down. She felt cold and sick. Her eyes were shut tight, but she could still see the terrible water and Pa's brown beard drowning in it. For a long, long time the wagon swayed and swung, and Mary cried without making a sound, and Laura's stomach felt sicker and sicker. Then the front wheels struck and grated, and Pa shouted. The whole wagon jerked and jolted and tipped backward, but the wheels were turning on the ground. Laura was up again, holding to the seat; she saw Pet's and Patty's scrambling wet backs climbing a steep bank, and Pa running beside them, shouting, 'Hi, Patty! Hi, Pet! Get up! Get up! Whoopsy-daisy! Good girls!

Laura reflects at the end of this extract that if Ma had not known what to do and if she and her sister had been naughty and bothered her, the whole family would have been swept away, their fate undiscovered until the next wagon went by, maybe weeks later. That would have been us, I fear.

ONCE, AT THE FOLK MUSEUM in Glencoe, my son, then aged about seven, dragged me over to a tableau showing a tartan-clad Alan Breck Stewart with his swordstick drawn while some waxwork ladies sat by the fireside with a plate of scones. Pointing to the text under the display, he asked me how these old ladies had kidnapped this man. Of course, Robert Louis Stevenson's *Kidnapped*, first published in 1886, is a stirring tale of Jacobites escaping through the heather. It was once widely read but has now fallen out of favour, probably because the writing is a bit flowery with many asides in the original. It's a cracking story, still.

'A sea-bred boy would not have stayed a day on Earraid.'
Kidnapped by Robert Louis Stevenson[23]

At the sudden tilting of the ship I was cast clean over the bulwarks into the sea. I went down, and drank my fill, and then came up, and got a blink of the moon, and then down again. They say a man sinks a third time for good. I cannot be made like other folk, then; for I would not like to write how often I went down, or how often I came up again. Presently, I found I was holding to a spar, which helped me somewhat. And then all of a sudden I was in quiet water, and began to come to myself. Hard work it was, and mortally slow; but in about an hour of kicking and splashing, I had got well in between the points of a sandy bay surrounded by low hills.

The sea was here quite quiet; there was no sound of any surf; the moon shone clear; and I thought in my heart I had never seen a place so desert and desolate. But it was dry land; and when at last it grew so shallow that I could wade ashore upon my feet, I cannot tell if I was more tired or more grateful.

With my stepping ashore I began the most unhappy part of my adventures. It was half-past twelve in the morning, and though the wind was broken by the land, it was a cold night. I dared not sit down (for I thought I should have frozen), but took off my shoes and walked to and fro upon the sand, bare-foot, and beating my breast with infinite weariness.

After a little, my way was stopped by a creek or inlet of the sea, which seemed to run pretty deep into the land; At first the creek kept narrowing but presently to my surprise it began to widen out again. At this I scratched my head, but had still no notion of the truth: until at last I came to a rising ground, and it burst upon me all in a moment that I was cast upon a little barren isle, and cut off on every side by the salt seas . . .

There is a pretty high rock on the northwest of Earraid. I was lying upon this rock on the third morning of this horrible life when all of a sudden, a coble with a brown sail and a pair of fishers aboard of it, came flying round that corner of the isle, bound for Iona. I shouted out, and then fell on my knees on the rock and reached up my hands and prayed to them. They were near enough to hear—I could even see the colour of their hair; and there was no doubt but they observed me, for they cried out in the Gaelic tongue, and laughed. But the boat never turned aside, and flew on, right before my eyes, for Iona.

I could not believe such wickedness, and ran along the shore from rock to rock, crying on them piteously even after they were out of reach of my voice, I still cried and waved to them; and when they were quite gone, I thought my heart would have burst. If a wish would kill men, those two fishers would never have seen morning, and I should likely have died upon my island.

The next day I found my bodily strength run very low. But the sun shone, the air was sweet. I was scarce back on my rock before I observed a boat coming down the Sound, and with her head, as I thought, in my direction.

I began at once to hope and fear; for I thought these men might have thought better of their cruelty and be coming back to my assistance. But another disappointment, such as yesterday's, was more than I could bear. I turned my back, accordingly, upon the sea, and did not look again till I had counted many hundreds. The boat was still heading for the island. The next time I counted the full thousand, as slowly as I could, my heart beating so as to hurt me. And then it was out of all question. She was coming straight to Earraid!

I could no longer hold myself back, but ran to the seaside and out, from one rock to another, as far as I could go. All this time the boat was coming on; and now I was able to perceive it was the same boat and the same two men as yesterday. This I knew by their hair, which the one had of a bright yellow and the other black. But now there was a third man along with them, who looked to be of a better class.

As soon as they were come within easy speech, they let down their sail and lay quiet. In spite of my supplications, they drew no nearer in, and what frightened me most of all, the new man tee-hee'd with laughter as he talked and looked at me. Then he stood up in the boat and addressed me a long while, speaking fast and with many wavings of his hand. I told him I had no Gaelic; and at this he became very angry, and I began to suspect he thought he was talking English. Listening very close, I caught the word 'whateffer' several times; but all the rest was Gaelic and might have been Greek and Hebrew for me.

'Whatever,' said I, to show him I had caught a word.

'Yes, yes—yes, yes,' says he, and then he looked at the other men, as much as to say, 'I told you I spoke English,' and began again as hard as ever in the Gaelic. This time I picked out another word, 'tide'. Then I had a flash of hope. I remembered he was always waving his hand towards the mainland of the Ross.

'Do you mean when the tide is out—?' I cried, and could not finish.

'Yes, yes,' said he. 'Tide.'

At that I turned tail upon their boat (where my adviser had once more begun to tee-hee with laughter), leaped back the way I had come, from one stone to another, and set off running across the isle as I had never run before. In about half an hour I came out upon the shores of the creek; and, sure enough, it was shrunk into a little trickle of water, through which I dashed, not above my knees, and landed with a shout on the main island.

A sea-bred boy would not have stayed a day on Earraid; which is only what they call a tidal islet, and except in the bottom of the neaps, can be entered and left twice in every twenty-four hours, either dry-shod, or at the most by wading.

CHAPTER VI

Adults at Play

OVER THE PAST SEVEN YEARS I've spent a lot of hours interviewing people who wild swim, for a series of books delving into the culture, and one theme that has repeatedly bubbled up is that adults will describe swimming as an act of play, or say that it's like 'getting to be a child again'.

Playing in water is actually what I think a lot of swimming is about – and it can link us to those early days of childhood. At Portobello beach, when I first started dipping with the community, I saw a lot of this silliness at work. Handstands in the shallows, post-swim conga dances, fancy-dress swims and even the Fife salute, a whipping off of a swim top to bare breasts towards the hills known as the Paps of Fife. We humans, I learned through looking at the research (as if I needed to be told), are neotenous creatures – we play throughout our adult lives.

It's as if, in the water, we reconnect to the sometimes lost current linking us to our childhood. The inner child is reinvigorated by a brisk, crashing wave. One splash and the decades wash away.

Many novels feature scenes of adults at play in the water, larking about as any child might do. Pulitzer-winner Richard Powers's 2024 work of fiction, *The Playground*, follows an oceanographer whose chief play is done in the magical undersea world in which she dives. It's there in other art forms too: a giddy verse, for instance, in Loudon Wainright III's humorous 'The Swimming Song', where he recalls a summer spent doing swan dives, jackknives and even 'a cannonball' into water.

One of the swimmers I often think of when it comes to the importance of play is Edinburgh dipper Christine Bell, a lawyer with a serious and challenging job who told me how swimming evokes 'the sensation of childhood'. Her story was echoed by many others.

'Swimming taps into a desire for adventure and playfulness.'

'Out to Play', from *Taking the Plunge* by Vicky Allan and Anna Deacon[24]

Christine, professor of law, Edinburgh

When people ask me when I started wild swimming, I sometimes say a couple of years ago, but the real answer is I've done it all my life. I've always swum. We lived in Derry, and, as a child, I spent all my summers in Donegal – right up on the most northerly point of Ireland. Because of the conflict, it was quite a magical place for me. We went swimming and I found I could go later and later in the year. I found that there were often really big waves at the equinox in October, which was our half-term break, and that the sea was really quite warm.

I have six children and a job that is very full on. I'm a Professor of Constitutional Law, and a lot of my work involves conflict and post-conflict situations. At the minute I run a big research programme which involves five different organisations. We look at how countries use the peace process to address issues of equality and inclusion. It's a career that has partly come out of the fact that I did a lot of human rights activism in the end days of the peace process in Northern Ireland.

My life is a bit impossible. I can't really take off into the mountains that easily – I can, but it needs a lot of planning and for the stars to align on the family front. But I can get down to the water here, and somehow if you go into the water you are in the wild. It's also very social going in with people.

For me, it probably relates to that sensation of childhood. We don't play enough as adults. I've often thought, why not? If we want to get fit, we go to gyms and go on treadmills which historically were torture instruments. But I was always fit and healthy as a child because I went out and played.

I can't hold down a regular commitment, but because you can arrange to swim an hour before and then be with people, it works for me. I like the spontaneity. Play is important. I see myself as quite serious; I'm quite driven and intense about my work. But having said that, humour is vital to me. I do try to have fun, even with our research team. It was a coping mechanism growing up: there was a very dark sort of humour around the Troubles. Banter and craic and humour are part of the culture of Ireland and Northern Ireland, and that's the case for me too. Swimming taps into a desire for adventure and playfulness.

~~~~~

IT IS NOT ALWAYS EASY, though, to find your inner child. Sometimes the interior grumpy old boy or girl will surface and complain about sand in the sandwiches or a bone-chilling east wind. *Three Men in a Boat (To Say Nothing of the Dog)* is a witty account of a boat journey by three friends on the Thames from Kingston upon Thames to Oxford and back. First published in 1889, it is the original lads' holiday. Here, the narrator Jerome writes about how his intention to bathe joyfully is sometimes quelled by the various discomforts of the seashore.

'They take the sea and put it two miles out.'

Three Men in a Boat by Jerome K. Jerome[25]

It is the same when you go to the sea-side. I always determine—when thinking over the matter in London—that I'll get up early every morning, and go and have a dip before breakfast, and I religiously pack up a pair of drawers and a bath towel. I always get red bathing drawers. I rather fancy myself in red drawers. They suit my complexion so. But when I get to the sea I don't feel somehow that I want that early morning bathe nearly so much as I did when I was in town.

On the contrary, I feel more that I want to stop in bed till the last moment, and then come down and have my breakfast. Once or twice virtue has triumphed, and I have got out at six and half-dressed myself, and have taken my drawers and towel, and stumbled dismally off. But I haven't enjoyed it. They seem to keep a specially cutting east wind, waiting for me, when I go to bathe in the early morning; and they pick out all the three-cornered stones, and put them on the top, and they sharpen up the rocks and cover the points over with a bit of sand so that I can't see them, and they take the sea and put it two miles out, so that I have to huddle myself up in my arms and hop, shivering, through six inches of water. And when I do get to the sea, it is rough and quite insulting.

One huge wave catches me up and chucks me in a sitting posture, as hard as ever it can, down on to a rock which has been put there for me. And, before I've said 'Oh! Ugh!' and found out what has gone, the wave comes back and carries me out to mid-ocean. I begin to strike out frantically for the shore, and wonder if I shall ever see home and friends again, and wish I'd been kinder to my little sister when a boy (when I was a boy, I mean). Just when I have given up all hope, a wave retires and leaves me sprawling like a star-fish on the sand, and I get up and look back and find that I've been swimming for my life in two feet of water. I hop back and dress, and crawl home, where I have to pretend I liked it.

In the present instance, we all talked as if we were going to have a long swim every morning.

George said it was so pleasant to wake up in the boat in the fresh morning, and plunge into the limpid river. Harris said there was nothing like a swim before breakfast to give you an appetite. He said it always gave him an appetite. George said that if it was going to make Harris eat more than Harris ordinarily ate, then he should protest against Harris having a bath at all. He said there would be quite enough hard work in towing sufficient food for Harris up against stream, as it was.

I urged upon George, however, how much pleasanter it would be to have Harris clean and fresh about the boat, even if we did have to take a few more hundredweight of provisions; and he got to see it in my light, and withdrew his opposition to Harris's bath.

Agreed, finally, that we should take *three* bath towels, so as not to keep each other waiting.

For clothes, George said two suits of flannel would be sufficient, as we could wash them ourselves, in the river, when they got dirty. We asked him if he had ever tried washing flannels in the river, and he replied: 'No, not exactly himself like; but he knew some fellows who had, and it was easy enough;' and Harris and I were weak enough to fancy he knew what he was talking about, and that three respectable young men, without position or influence, and with no experience in washing, could really clean their own shirts and trousers in the river Thames with a bit of soap.

We were to learn in the days to come, when it was too late, that George was a miserable impostor, who could evidently have known nothing whatever about the matter. If you had seen these clothes after— but, as the shilling shockers say, we anticipate.

～

JACK LONDON, ADVENTUROUS AUTHOR OF *Call of the Wild*, seems, at least in his muscular prose, like the kind of guy who would always relish a bathe in rough seas. In this section from 'The Kanaka Surf', a short story from the turn of the twentieth century, we are treated to an inspiring description of an intrepid and beautiful couple, Ida and Lee, catching a big wave.

'On and up, to the sprouting beard of growing crest, the colour orgy.'
'The Kanaka Surf' by Jack London[26]

The captain suddenly sprang upon the railing of the lanai, held on to a pillar with one hand, and again picked up the two specks of heads through the glasses. His surprise was verified. The two fools had veered out of the channel toward Diamond Head, and were directly seaward of the kanaka surf. Worse, as he looked, they were starting to come in through the kanaka surf . . .

The captain saw the first kanaka wave, large of itself, but small among its fellows, lift seaward behind the two speck-swimmers. Then he saw them strike a crawl-stroke, side by side, faces downward, full-lengths out-stretched on surface, their feet sculling like propellers and their arms flailing in rapid over-hand strokes, as they spurted speed to approximate the speed of the overtaking wave, so that, when overtaken, they would become part of the wave, and travel with it instead of being left behind it. Thus, if they were coolly skilled enough to ride outstretched on the surface and the forward face of the crest instead of being flung and crumpled or driven head-first to bottom, they would dash shoreward, not propelled by their own energy, but by the energy of the wave into which they had become incorporated.

And they did it! 'SOME swimmers!' the captain of Number Nine made the announcement to himself under his breath. He continued to gaze eagerly. The best of swimmers could hold such a wave for several hundred feet. But could they? If they did, they would be a third of the way through the perils they had challenged. But, not unexpected by him, the woman failed first, her body not presenting the larger surfaces that her husband's did. At the end of seventy feet she was overwhelmed, being driven downward and out of sight by the tons of water in the over-topple. Her husband followed and both appeared swimming beyond the wave they had lost.

The captain saw the next wave first. 'If they try to body-surf on that, good night,' he muttered; for he knew the swimmer did not live who would tackle it. Beardless itself, it was father of all bearded ones, a mile long, rising up far out beyond where the others rose, towering its solid bulk higher and higher till it blotted out the horizon, and was a giant among its fellows ere its beard began to grow as it thinned its crest to the over-curl.

But it was evident that the man and woman knew big water. No racing stroke did they make in advance of the wave. The captain inwardly applauded as he saw them turn and face the wave and wait for it. It was a picture that of all on the beach he alone saw, wonderfully distinct and vivid in the magnification of the binoculars. The wall of the wave was truly a wall, mounting, ever mounting, and thinning, far up, to a transparency of the colours of the setting sun shooting athwart all the green and blue of it. The green thinned to lighter green that merged blue even as he looked. But it was a blue gem-brilliant with innumerable sparkle-points of rose and gold flashed through it by the sun. On and up, to the sprouting beard of growing crest, the colour orgy increased until it was a kaleidoscopic effervescence of transfusing rainbows.

Against the face of the wave showed the heads of the man and woman like two sheer specks. Specks they were, of the quick, adventuring among the blind elemental forces, daring the titanic buffets of the sea. The weight of the down-fall of that father of waves, even then imminent above their heads, could stun a man or break the fragile bones of a woman. The captain of Number Nine was unconscious that he was holding his breath. He was oblivious of the man. It was the woman. Did she lose her head or courage, or misplay her muscular part for a moment, she could be hurled a hundred feet by that giant buffet and left wrenched, helpless, and breathless to be pulped on the coral bottom and sucked out by the undertow to be battened on by the fish-sharks too cowardly to take their human meat alive.

Why didn't they dive deep, and with plenty of time, the captain wanted to know, instead of waiting till the last tick of safety and the first tick of peril were one? He saw the woman turn her head and laugh to the man, and his head turn in response. Above them, overhanging them, as they mounted the body of the wave, the beard, creaming white, then frothing into rose and gold, tossed upward into a spray of jewels. The crisp off-shore trade-wind caught the beard's fringes and blew them backward and upward yards and yards into the air. It was then, side by side, and six feet apart, that they dived straight under the over-curl even then disintegrating to chaos and falling. Like insects disappearing into the convolutions of some gorgeous gigantic orchid, so they disappeared, as beard and crest and spray and jewels, in many tons, crashed and thundered down just where they had disappeared the moment before, but where they were no longer.

Beyond the wave they had gone through, they finally showed, side by side, still six feet apart, swimming shoreward with a steady stroke until the next wave should make them body-surf it or face and pierce it. The captain of Number Nine waved his hand to his crew in dismissal, and sat down on the lanai railing, feeling vaguely tired and still watching the swimmers through his glasses.

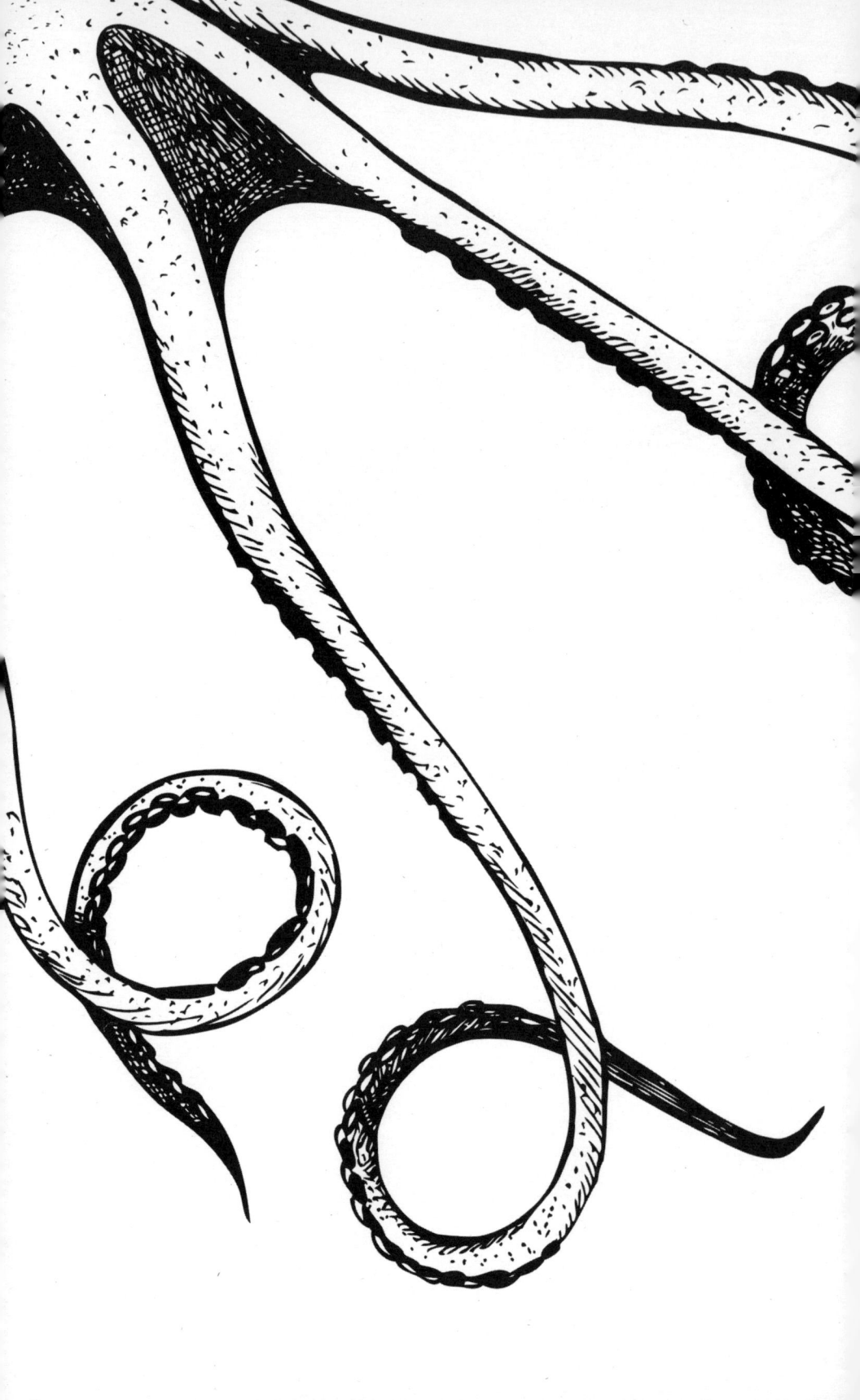

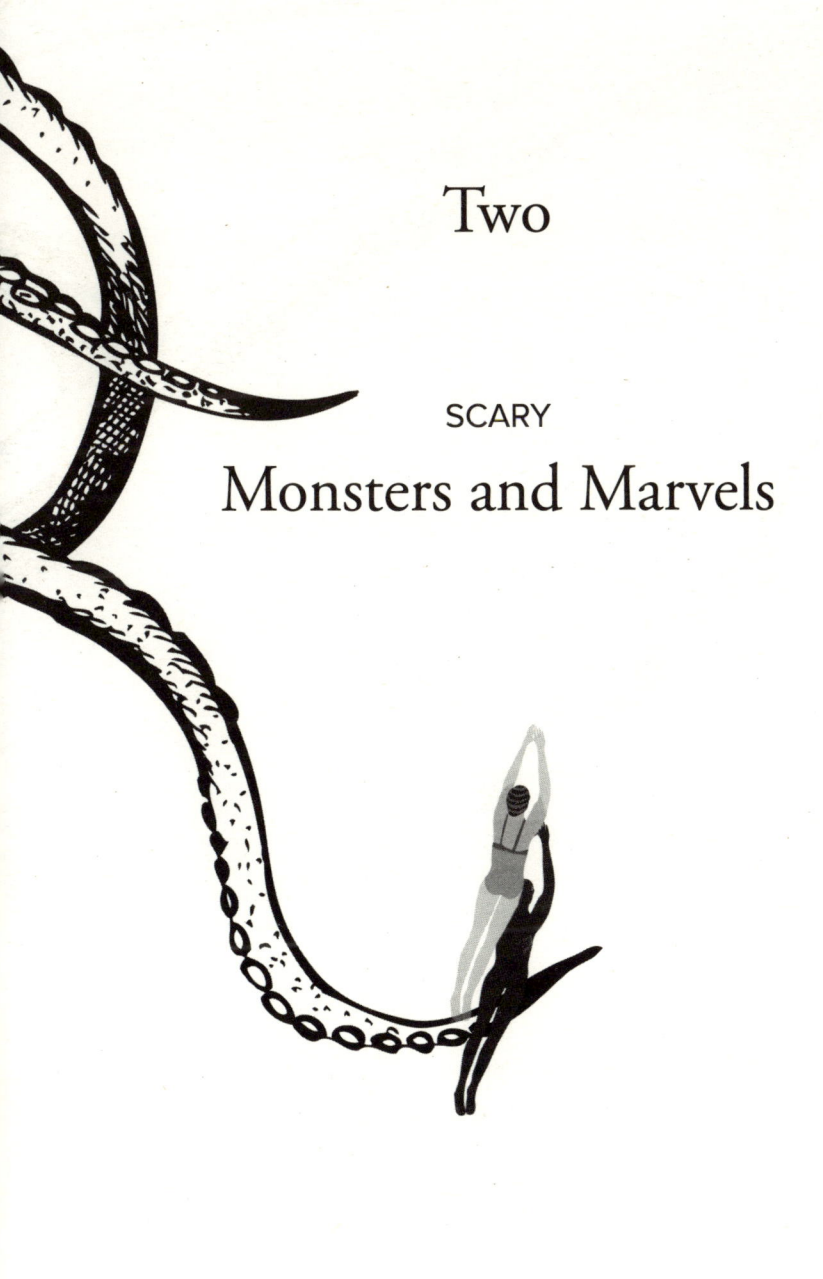

Two

SCARY

Monsters and Marvels

IT'S NOT, MANY SWIMMERS WILL say, the water they fear, but what lies beneath. The snaggle-toothed pike lurking in the lake; the jellyfish drifting near the shore; the shark's fin piercing the surface; the brittle claw tickling at one's toes.

Above all, though, it's the thing unknown. For the sea is not just a realm of cod, haddock and common crab, but of the strange and alien. The unpredictable and unseen. It's home to serpents and monsters, unimaginable creatures of the deep.

The most profound waters – the midnight zone and the abyss – really are, as photographs testify, home to forms weird and uncanny, the truly other. We swimmers don't tend to come close to these, but for our imaginations it's enough to know they are somewhere down there.

Of course, many of the strange and wonderful creatures who really do inhabit the deep, from hammerhead sharks to the tiny polyps that make up coral reefs are now endangered. Which begs the question, when it comes to the sea, who is the real monster?

CHAPTER I

See Monsters

SWIMMING IS PARTLY ABOUT CONFRONTING our fear of those monsters – the creatures that nip, slither, brush past us and bite. It can also, through the window of goggles or a mask, be about marvelling at their beauty, finding wonder – and knowledge – in a world that is so very different from our own.

Deep waters can bring to the surface the monsters of our own psyche. I remember being struck, as a young woman, reading Iris Murdoch's 1978 novel *The Sea, The Sea*, by how she captured that experience of having glimpsed something monstrous, and the lingering uncertainty over its reality.

A scene featuring a vision of such a serpent or monster got me hooked on the author's writing, and on the idea of wild swimming around Britain's rugged coves. In *The Sea, The Sea*, the abominable Charles Arrowby, a theatre director and bully, has taken himself off to a cottage to write his memoirs and, while there, indulges in some naked swimming. One day, looking down from the cliffs into the rolling waters of the ocean, he catches sight of a terrifying vision.

**'As my eyes became accustomed to the glare,
I saw a monster rising from the waves.'**
The Sea, The Sea by Iris Murdoch[27]

I went swimming again but still cannot discover quite the right place. This morning I simply dived into deep water off the rocks nearest to the house, where they descend almost sheer, yet with folds and ledges enough to make precarious stairway. My 'cliff' I call it, though it is barely twenty feet high at low tide. Of course the water is very cold, but after a few seconds it seems to coat the body in kind of warm silvery skin, as if one had acquired the scales of a merman. The challenged blood rejoices with a new strength. Yes, this is my natural element. How strange to think that I never saw the sea until I was fourteen.

I am a skilful fearless swimmer and I am not afraid of rough water. Today the sea was gentle compared with antipodean oceans where I have sported like a dolphin. My problem was almost a technical one. Even though the swell was fairly mild I had a ridiculous amount of difficulty getting back onto the rocks again. The 'cliff' was a little too steep, the ledges a little too narrow. The gentle waves teased me, lifting me up towards the rock face, then plucking me away. My fingers, questing for a crevice, were again and again pulled off. Becoming tired, I swam around trying other places where the sea was running restlessly in and out, but the difficulty was greater since there was deep water below me and even if the rocks were less sheer they were smoother or slippery with weed and I could not hold on. At last I managed to climb up my cliff, clinging with fingers and toes, then kneeling sideways upon a ledge. When I reached the top and lay panting in the sun I found that my hands and knees were bleeding.

Since my arrival I have had the pleasure of swimming naked. This rocky coast attracts, thank God, no trippers with their kiddies. There is not a vestige of beastly sand anywhere. I have heard it called an ugly coast. Long may it be deemed so. The rocks, which stretch away in both directions, are not in fact picturesque. They are sandy yellow in colour, covered with crystalline flecks, and are folded into large ungainly incoherent heaps. Below the tide line they are festooned with growths of glistening blistery dark brown seaweed which has a rather unpleasant smell. Up above however, and at close quarters, they afford the clamberer a surprising number of secret joys.

Some pages on, he describes a memory of a strange and terrifying sight in the water:

I was sitting, with this notebook beside me, upon the rocks just above my 'cliff', and looking out over the water. The sun was shining, the sea was calm. (As I have described it in the first paragraph of this notebook.) Shortly before this I had been looking intently into a rock pool and watching a remarkably long reddish faintly bristly sea worm which had wreathed itself into curious coils prior to disappearing into a hole. I sat up, then settled myself facing seaward, blinking in the sun. Then, not at once, but after about two minutes, as my eyes became accustomed to the glare, I saw a monster rising from the waves.

I can describe this in no other way. Out of a perfectly calm empty sea, at a distance of perhaps a quarter of a mile (or less), I saw an immense creature break the surface and arch itself upward. At first it looked like a black snake, then a long thickening body with a ridgy spiny back followed the elongated neck. There was something which might have been a flipper or perhaps a fin. I could not see the whole of the creature, but the remainder of its body, or perhaps a long tail, disturbed the foaming water round the base of what had now risen from the sea to a height of (as it seemed) twenty or thirty feet. The creature then coiled itself so that the long neck circled twice, bringing the now conspicuous head low down above the surface of the sea. I could see the sky through the coils. I could also see the head with remarkable clarity, a kind of crested snake's head, green-eyed, the mouth opening to show teeth and a pink interior. The head and neck glistened with a blue sheen. Then in a moment the whole thing collapsed, the coils fell, the undulating back still broke the water, and then there was nothing but a great foaming swirling pool where the creature had vanished.

The shock and the horror of it were so great that for some time I could not move. I wanted to run away, I feared beyond anything that the animal would reappear closer to land, perhaps rising up at my very feet. But my legs would not function and my heart was beating so violently that any further exertion might have rendered me unconscious. The sea had become calm again and nothing further happened. At last I got up and walked slowly back to the house. I went up the stairs and into the drawing room where I sat for some time just breathing carefully and holding my heart. I could not bear to take my usual place at the window, so I sat at the little table against the wall of the inner room, leaning my head against the wall, and about half an hour later I was able to write down what now appears as the second paragraph in this notebook.

During that time, as I held on to myself and breathed and trembled, I managed gradually to think about what had occurred. Thought, rational thought, which had been utterly routed, returned gradually to my rescue.

Something had happened and happenings have explanations. Several possible explanations came before me, and as I began to number and classify and relate them some relief came, and the awful unconceptualised terror receded. It was possible that I had 'simply' imagined what I saw. But of course one does not 'simply' imagine anything so detailed and dreadful. It later struck me as significant that the creature had appeared at once as utterly frightful, rather than as very surprising or even interesting. I was excessively frightened. I am a moderate drinker and certainly not an unbalanced or crazily 'imaginative' person.

Another possibility was that I had, again 'simply', seen a monster unknown to science. Well, that was just possible. Or: was what I had seen an absolutely enormous eel? Could there be such an eel? Did eels ever rise up out of the sea and wreathe themselves into coils and balance themselves high in the air? I could not think that the thing was an eel, this was impossible. It had a substantial body, I had seen its back. I was quite sure too that I could not have seen a mere eel, however large, as this coiling monstrosity through which I had looked at the sky.

How far off had the animal been and how high above the water had it risen? On further reflection I was not so certain of my first impressions, though I remained sure that I had seen something absolutely remarkable.

Explanations in terms of floating seaweed or bobbing driftwood were not to be considered. I explored another possibility. Just before I saw my huge monster I had been closely inspecting, in the rock pool, a little monster, the red bristling worm, whose five or six inches of wriggling body appeared big in the confined space of the pool. Was it possible that through some purely optical mechanism, some unusual trick of the retina, I had 'thrown' the image of the worm out onto the surface of the sea? This was an interesting idea but totally implausible, since the red worm bore no resemblance to the bluish-blackish monster, except in so far as both of them had wreathed into coils. Besides, I had never heard of any such retinal 'cinematography'. I was struck, on reflection, by the fact that I recalled the creature with extreme clarity, the visual impression remained extremely detailed, while at the same time I felt more and more vague about its exact distance away from me.

ULTIMATELY CHARLES ARROWBY BLAMES HIS vision on LSD, and the reigniting of a 'bad trip' from his past. His experience, whether drug-induced or some other conjuring, seems to tap into a wider cultural consciousness.

Our literature and mythology is brim-full of sea monsters. They have slipped and slithered their way through countless writings throughout history.

Beowulf, first written down in the Middle Ages but from a far older oral tradition, is about the warrior defeating a monster called Grendel who lives in the swamps. During a dispute about whether Beowulf is man enough for the challenge, he is accused of having once lost a swimming match against his friend Breca. The hero retaliates by explaining that, during the swim, he had to take constant breaks to slay sea fiends.

'A hateful fiend-scather, seized me and held me.'

Beowulf, translated by John Lesslie Hall[28]

> We made agreement as the merest of striplings
> Promised each other (both of us then were
> Younkers in years) that we two would venture
> Out on the waves;
> Then we as companions stayed in the ocean
> Five nights together, till the currents did part us,
> The weltering waters, the weather the bleakest,
> At night's darkest reaches, with the north-wind whistling
> Fierce in our faces; strong were the billows.

A hateful fiend-scather, seized me and held me,
To the bottom then dragged me,
Grimly we grappled, then was I able
To pierce the monster with the point of my weapon,
My obedient blade carried away
The mighty mere-creature by means of my hand-blow

~

GERMAN PLAYWRIGHT FRIEDRICH SCHILLER'S LATE eighteenth-century ballad 'The Diver' features another heroic monster-wrangler. The tale was apparently inspired by a legendary swimmer who had webbed hands and feet. Challenged by the king to dive into the deep after a golden cup, a brave page glimpses an abyss full of fish and, among them, a huge monster.

'Then a *something* crawled near.'
'The Diver' by Friedrich Schiller[29]

'What knight or what vassal will be so bold
As to plunge in the gulf below?
See! I hurl in its depths a goblet of gold,
Already the waters over it flow.
The man who can bring back the goblet to me,
May keep it henceforward,—his own it shall be.'

All before him in silence stand,
When a page, with a modest pride,
Steps out of the timorous squirely band,
And his girdle and mantle soon throws aside . . .

91

The young man waits for a break in the waves and plunges in.

Then quickly, before the breakers rebound,
The stripling commends him to Heaven,
And—a scream of horror is heard around,—
As now by the whirlpool away he is taken,
And closely over the swimmer brave
Close the jaws, and he vanishes 'neath the dark wave . . .

Eventually the young man re-emerges holding the goblet. The king's beautiful daughter fills it with sparkling wine, and the youth recounts what he saw:

'I was torn below with the speed of light,
When out of a cavern of rock
Rushed towards me a spring with furious might;
I was seized by the sudden torrent's wild shock,
And like a top, with a whirl and a bound,
Despite all resistance, was whirled around.

'Then God pointed out,—for to Him I cried
In that terrible moment of need,—
A craggy reef in the gulf's dark side;
I seized it in haste, and from death was then freed.

'And there, on sharp corals, was hanging the cup,—
The fathomless pit had else swallowed it up . . .
'There crowded, in union fearful and black,

In a horrible mass entwined,
The rock-fish, the ray with the thorny back,
And the hammer-fish's misshapen kind,
And the shark, the hyena dread of the sea,
With his angry teeth, grinned fiercely on me.

'Then a *something* crawled near,
And a hundred limbs out-flung,
And at me it snapped;—in my mortal fear,
I left hold of the coral to which I had clung;
Then the whirlpool seized on me with maddened roar,
Yet 'twas well, for it brought me to light once more.'

Unfortunately for the hero, the king demands he return and swim into the abyss to report on what he finds down there: he does so and is never seen again.

~~~

SOMETIMES WHO THE MONSTER IS, is a question of perspective, as this passage in *Alice's Adventures in Wonderland* suggests.

'I wish I hadn't cried so much!'
Alice's Adventures in Wonderland by Lewis Carroll[30]

'That *WAS* a narrow escape!' said Alice, a good deal frightened at the sudden change, but very glad to find herself still in existence; 'and now for the garden!' and she ran with all speed back to the little door: but, alas! the little door was shut again, and the little golden key was lying on the glass table as before, 'and things are worse than ever,' thought the poor child, 'for I never was so small as this before, never! And I declare it's too bad, that it is!'

As she said these words her foot slipped, and in another moment, splash! she was up to her chin in salt water. He first idea was that she had somehow fallen into the sea, 'and in that case I can go back by railway,' she said to herself. (Alice had been to the seaside once in her life, and had come to the general conclusion, that wherever you go to on the English coast you find a number of bathing machines in the sea, some children digging in the sand with wooden spades, then a row of lodging houses, and behind them a railway station.) However, she soon made out that she was in the pool of tears which she had wept when she was nine feet high.

'I wish I hadn't cried so much!' said Alice, as she swam about, trying to find her way out. 'I shall be punished for it now, I suppose, by being drowned in my own tears! That will be a queer thing, to be sure! However, everything is queer to-day.'

Just then she heard something splashing about in the pool a little way off, and she swam nearer to make out what it was: at first she thought it must be a walrus or hippopotamus, but then she remembered how small she was now, and she soon made out that it was only a mouse that had slipped in like herself.

'Would it be of any use, now,' thought Alice, 'to speak to this mouse? Everything is so out-of-the-way down here, that I should think very likely it can talk: at any rate, there's no harm in trying.' So she began: 'O Mouse, do you know the way out of this pool? I am very tired of swimming about here, O Mouse!' (Alice thought this must be the right way of speaking to a mouse: she had never done such a thing before, but she remembered having seen in her brother's Latin Grammar,

'A mouse — of a mouse — to a mouse — a mouse — O mouse!' The Mouse looked at her rather inquisitively, and seemed to her to wink with one of its little eyes, but it said nothing.

'Perhaps it doesn't understand English,' thought Alice; 'I daresay it's a French mouse, come over with William the Conqueror.' (For, with all her knowledge of history, Alice had no very clear notion how long ago anything had happened.) So she began again: 'Ou est ma chatte?' which was the first sentence in her French lesson-book. The Mouse gave a sudden leap out of the water, and seemed to quiver all over with fright. 'Oh, I beg your pardon!' cried Alice hastily, afraid that she had hurt the poor animal's feelings. 'I quite forgot you didn't like cats.'

'Not like cats!' cried the Mouse, in a shrill, passionate voice. 'Would *you* like cats if you were me?'

'Well, perhaps not,' said Alice in a soothing tone: 'don't be angry about it. And yet I wish I could show you our cat Dinah: I think you'd take a fancy to cats if you could only see her. She is such a dear quiet thing,' Alice went on, half to herself, as she swam lazily about in the pool, 'and she sits purring so nicely by the fire, licking her paws and washing her face — and she is such a nice soft thing to nurse — and she's such a capital one for catching mice — oh, I beg your pardon!' cried Alice again, for this time the Mouse was bristling all over, and she felt certain it must be really offended. 'We won't talk about her any more if you'd rather not.'

'We indeed!' cried the Mouse, who was trembling down to the end of his tail. 'As if I would talk on such a subject! Our family always *hated* cats: nasty, low, vulgar things! Don't let me hear the name again!'

'I won't indeed!' said Alice, in a great hurry to change the subject of conversation. 'Are you — are you fond — of — of dogs?' The Mouse did not answer, so Alice went on eagerly: 'There is such a nice little dog near our house I should like to show you! A little bright-eyed terrier, you know, with oh, such long curly brown hair! And it'll fetch things when you throw them, and it'll sit up and beg for its dinner, and all sorts of things – I can't remember half of them – and it belongs to a farmer, you know, and he says it's so useful, it's worth a hundred pounds! He says it kills all the rats and – oh dear!' cried Alice in a sorrowful tone, 'I'm afraid I've offended it again!' For the Mouse was swimming away from her as hard as it could go, and making quite a commotion in the pool as it went.

So she called softly after it, 'Mouse dear! Do come back again, and we won't talk about cats or dogs either, if you don't like them!' When the Mouse heard this, it turned round and swam slowly back to her: its face was quite pale (with passion, Alice thought), and it said in a low trembling voice, 'Let us get to the shore, and then I'll tell you my history, and you'll understand why it is I hate cats and dogs.'

It was high time to go, for the pool was getting quite crowded with the birds and animals that had fallen into it: there were a Duck and a Dodo, a Lory and an Eaglet, and several other curious creatures. Alice led the way, and the whole party swam to the shore.

CHAPTER II

Marvellous Sea Creatures

NOT ALWAYS ARE WATER MONSTERS simply the creations of human imagination. Sometimes they are the marvels of actual marine life. The fourteenth-century Arabian explorer Ibn Battuta travelled further than any of his contemporaries. Near the end of his life, he dictated an account of his journeys, in which Battuta encounters some astonishing beasts.

'Their heads are like horses' heads, and their feet are like elephants' feet.'
A Gift to Those Who Contemplate the Wonders of Cities and the Marvels of Travelling by Ibn Battuta[31]

When we reached the channel, I saw on the bank sixteen beasts with huge bodies. I wondered at them and supposed they were elephants, which are numerous there. Then I saw they had gone into the river. I said to Abū Bakr b. Ya'qūb: 'What are these beasts?' He said: 'They are hippopotamuses which have come out to graze on land.' They are bigger than horses, they have manes and tails, their heads are like horses' heads, and their feet are like elephants' feet. I saw them another time when I was sailing on the Nile from Tunbuktū to Kawkaw. They swim in the river and lift their heads and blow. The boatmen were afraid of them and drew near to land to avoid being drowned by them. They have an ingenious trick for hunting them. They have spears pierced with holes through which they put strong cords. They strike the hippopotamus with them and, if the blow strikes the foot or the neck it pierces right through and they pull on the rope till it comes to the bank when they kill the hippopotamus and eat the flesh. There are many of the bones lying on the bank.

~~~~~

DOLPHINS, WITH THEIR INTELLIGENCE, FACIAL expressions so like a human smile and irresistible piping cries, are beloved by people. Sadly, this does not always mean we treat them well. Even today, there is still money to be made out of bringing dolphins into captivity, offering the entertainment or therapy of riding or swimming with them. But we can nevertheless take pleasure in the story of a swim with a free-living cetacean – or this 2,000-year-old story of a singer-songwriter, riding atop a dolphin with a lyre.

Here in the Roman poet Ovid's book of festivals and feast days, *Fasti*, the constellation of the dolphin enters the water and takes on a supernatural role, saving the hero Arion from a robbery and murder plot.

'He could hold back the running waters with his singing.'
Fasti, Book II by Ovid[32]

The Dolphin that you saw lately, studded with stars,
Will escape your gaze on the following night:

He was a happy go-between in love's intrigues,
Or he carried the Lesbian lyre and its master.
What land or sea does not know of Arion?
He could hold back the running waters with his singing.
Often the wolf seeking a lamb was halted by his voice,
Often the lamb stopped, in fleeing the ravening wolf.
Often hare and hounds rested in the same covert,
And the deer on the rock stood still near the lioness,
And the chattering crow perched with Pallas' owl,
Without a quarrel, and the dove united with the hawk.
They say that Diana has often stood entranced at your music,
Tuneful Arion, as if it were played by her brother's hand.
Arion's fame had filled the cities of Sicily,
And charmed the Italian shores with the sound of his lyre:
Travelling back from there, he boarded a ship
Carrying with him the wealth won by his art.
Unhappy one, perhaps you feared the wind and waves,
But the sea, in truth, was safer for you than your ship.
Since the steersman stood there with naked blade,
And the rest of that crew of conspirators were armed.
Why draw that blade? Seaman, steer the wandering vessel:
That weapon is not appropriate in your hands.
Trembling with fear, Arion said: 'I don't plead for life,
But let me take up my lyre and play a little.'
They granted it, laughing at the delay. He took the wreath
That might have graced your tresses, Phoebus:
Put on his robe, twice-stained with Tyrian purple:
And, plucked by his thumb, the strings gave out their music,
Such a melody as the swan's mournful measures,

When the cruel shaft has transfixed its brow.
At once, he plunged, fully clothed into the waves:
The water, leaping, splashed the sky-blue stern.
Then (beyond belief) they say a dolphin
Yielded its back to the unaccustomed weight.
Sitting there, Arion gripped the lyre, and paid his fare
In song, soothing the ocean waves with his singing.
The gods see good deeds: Jupiter took the dolphin
And ordered its constellation to contain nine stars.

~~~

BUT ONE PARTICULAR REAL-LIFE MONSTER seems to haunt contemporary mythology more than any other. It has a theme tune, hard-wired into our minds like the sound of our own heartbeat quickening. It's there in the glimpse of something dark on the water, perhaps the unmistakable sharp line of a fin. Author Peter Benchley and director Steven Spielberg are the storytellers who carved the shape of that fear into our collective consciousness with the 1975 movie *Jaws*. Its title alone is like a synecdoche of terror.

For people who grew up in the late twentieth century, *Jaws* influenced our relationship with sharks, impacting on their conservation and, of course, the danger they posed in our imaginations. But the rogue shark theory that forms the dramatic lynchpin of *Jaws* has now been discredited and Benchley came to regret the war on these prehistoric predators that was intensified by the movie's blockbuster success. Of course, the reputation of the great white shark is not entirely fictional. These marine hunters, with an astonishing bite force among the strongest in the animal world, do sometimes kill, or terribly maim humans and those real-life stories, though rare, terrify us.

The predatory shark as an idea is older than *Jaws* – in the absurdist *Songs of Maldoror* by the Comte de Lautréamont, the killer beast meets her match in the evil narrator. This poetic story cycle, written in the mid-nineteenth century, but later rediscovered by the Surrealists and Symbolists, expresses the idea that there is one creature to be found in the sea who is more brutal and dangerous than any other – man.

'What is the army of sea-monsters cleaving the waves so rapidly?'
Songs of Maldoror by the Comte de Lautréamont[33]

I sought a soul akin to mine but I could not find one. I searched every corner of the earth; my perseverance brought no reward. Yet I could not remain alone. Someone had to approve of my character, someone had to have the same ideas as I.

A ship sinks and Maldoror takes a gun and shoots a survivor escaping the wreck. The ship then sinks completely.

I was not so cruel as men later made me out to be . . . but unfortunately on the night of the tempest, a fit of rage had come upon me, my reason had deserted me and I vowed that everything which fell into my hands that night would have to die.

When the dark circle where the vessel had been struggling clearly showed that it had gone to spend the rest of its days on the ground floor of the sea some of those who had been carried off by the waves began to appear on the surface, They held one another round the waist in twos and threes, it was a good way of not saving their lives; for their movements became entangled and they went down like leaking jugs. But what is the army of sea-monsters cleaving the waves so rapidly? There are three of them, their fins are strong and they are forcing their way through the heaving seas.

The sharks soon make only an omelette without eggs of all the human beings moving their limbs, and share it among themselves according to the law of the strongest. The blood mixes with the waters. Their wild eyes illuminate the scene of the carnage . . . But, what else is this tumult of the waters, over there, on the horizon? It looks like a typhoon approaching. What flailing! I see what it is.

A huge female shark comes to partake of the pâté de foie gras and cold beef. She is furious; because she is starving. A fight begins between her and the sharks, to compete for the few throbbing members that float here and there, silently, on the surface of the red cream. To the right, to the left, she launches bites which cause mortal wounds. But three living sharks still surround her, and she is forced to snap in all directions to foil their tricks. With swelling emotion, such as he has never felt, the spectator follows this new kind of naval battle from the shore. His eyes are fixed on this courageous female shark, with such strong teeth. He no longer hesitates, he shoulders his rifle, and, with his customary skill, he lodges his second bullet in the gills of one of the sharks, just as it appears above a wave.

There remain two sharks who, seeing this, go in even more eagerly. From the top of the rock, the man with the briny saliva throws himself into the sea, and swims towards the pleasantly coloured carpet, holding in his hand a steel knife which he always carries. Now every shark faces an enemy. He advances towards his tired adversary, and, taking his time, thrusts his sharp blade into his stomach. He easily gets rid of the last opponent . . .

The swimmer is now in the presence of the female shark he has saved. They looked into each other's eyes for a few minutes: each surprised to find so much ferocity in the other's eyes. They swim in circles, never losing sight of each other, and say to themselves: 'I have been wrong so far; here's one who's meaner.' Then, by mutual agreement, between two waters, they glide towards each other, with mutual admiration, the female shark parting the water with her fins, Maldoror beating the wave with his arms: and holding their breath, in deep reverence, each eager to contemplate, for the first time, his living portrait.

Arriving three meters apart, without making any effort, they suddenly fall upon each other, like two magnets, and embrace with dignity and gratitude. Carnal desires closely followed this demonstration of friendship. Two sinewy thighs cling tightly to the monster's viscous skin, like two leeches; and, the arms and fins intertwined around the body of the beloved object, while their throats and their chests soon became nothing more than a greyish mass amid the tendrils of seaweed; in the middle of the storm which continued to rage; in the light of lightning; having as their mating bed the foaming wave, carried away by an underwater current as in a cradle, and rolling on top of one another, towards the depths of the abyss, they unite in a long, chaste and hideous coupling!

Finally, I had found one akin to me! . . . From now on, I was no longer alone in life! . . . She had the same ideas as me! . . . I was face to face with my first love!

CHAPTER III
Monsters Are Us

SOME MYTHOLOGICAL SEA CREATURES ARE, of course, a little more like us. Halfway towards being human, and yet belonging to the sea or other waters, these are the instantly recognisable and alluring merfolk, selkies and water spirits.

Wild swimmers will sometimes talk about being mermaids, or feeling more merfolk or selkie than human when they swim – as if the act of submersion triggers some metamorphosis, delivering them up to some ancestral aquatic self. In *Taking the Plunge*, one swimmer told me how the selkie story had become important to them during gender transition. 'Selkies have another truer form that is not seen by land folk and I do too,' they said. 'It's also a really beautiful way of thinking about being at home in one's skin. When I swim outdoors, I feel free from the constraints of gender and societal expectations of my body – I am fluid and free; I feel at home in my skin.'

Some, like ice swimmer and Merthyr Mermaid, Cath Pendleton, or campaigner Lindsey Cole, like to don a fake – and sometimes glitteringly elaborate – tail. With a flip of a fabric monofin, they shapeshift and tap into a complex mythological history in poetry, prose and oral storytelling.

Selkies, often found in Scottish and Nordic folklore, are beings that can shift between human or seal form by removing or donning their sealskin. In a book called *Seal-folk and Ocean Paddlers: Sliochd Nan Ròn*, published in 1998, Hebridean boatbuilder John M. MacAuley explored the idea that the legends of selkies, the seal people, had a real basis in the Indigenous peoples of northern Scandinavia. They faced discrimination from the settlers in their lands, who became known to us as the Vikings, and may have drifted south to seek refuge. He thinks the legends could have been inspired by occasional visits from Sámi people, in sealskin kayaks and wearing sealskin garments. These sealskins, while practical at sea, would have needed to be dried out after prolonged time in the water, so it would not be impossible that a fisherman could have found a Sámi woman on a rock, drying her 'skin'.

In this Orkney ballad of Sule Skerry, the selkie is male.

'I am a selchie on the sea.'
Sule Skerry, Orkney ballad[34]

> I am a man upon the land;
> I am a selchie on the sea,
> and when I'm far frae ev'ry strand,
> my dwelling is in Sule Skerry.

~

ANOTHER SUCH TALE, RECORDED BY Orkney folklorist Walter Traill Dennison in the late nineteenth century, features Magnus, a fisherman who once rescued a selkie but later finds himself suddenly caught, while wading out to fish for coal-fish, by the incoming tide.

The fisherman, as the sea is coming round his throat, rippling into his mouth and lifting him away from the rock, finds himself gripped by the back of the neck by some being; he is saved by the selkie he once rescued.

'Summin' grippid him bae thc neck o' the co't an' whippid him aff o' his feet.'

The Selkie that Deud No' Forget by Walter Traill Dennison[35]

The water raise an' raise, cam' ap abeun his knees, abeun his henches, ap tae his oxters; an' miny a sair sich gae he, as de water cam' aye hicher an' nearer tae his chin. He cried whill he wus trapple-hers', an' he could cry nee mair. An' dan he gae ap; a' hup' o' life, an' saw naething afore him bit dismal daeth. An' dan, as de sea wus comin' roond his hass, an' comin' noos and dans i' peedie lippers tae his mooth, jeust as he f'and the sea beginnan' tae lift him fae the rock, – summin' grippid him bae thc neck o' the co't an' whippid him aff o' his feet. He kent no' what hid wus, or whar he wus, till he f'and his feet at the boddam whar he could wad ashore i' safety. An' whin de craeter 'at hed haud o' him passed him, he wadded tae the dry land.

~~~~~

THE GREAT IRISH POET W.B. Yeats also touched on this theme.

'A mermaid found a swimming lad.'

'A Man Young and Old: III. The Mermaid' by William Butler Yeats (from *The Tower*)[36]

A mermaid found a swimming lad,
Picked him for her own,

Pressed her body to his body,
Laughed; and plunging down
Forgot in cruel happiness
That even lovers drown.

～

SCIENCE FICTION WRITER H. G. WELLS delved into mermaid lore when he wrote his 1901 fantasy novel, *The Sea Lady*. Inspired by the sighting of a young woman he knew wearing a bathing suit, the satire starts with the arrival ashore of a social-climbing, romance-seeking mermaid at Sandgate. It exploits aspects of mermaid mythology as it examines societal norms, suffrage and the hypocrisies of Victorian life.

The action begins when a figure is spotted in the water and two gentlemen, described as not particularly 'expert swimmers', plunge in to her rescue.

"'Cramp," she said, "I have cramp." Both the men were convinced of that.'
The Sea Lady by H. G. Wells[37]

And then quite unexpectedly the Sea Lady appeared beside them. One lovely arm supported Mr. Bunting about the waist and the other was over the ladder. She did not appear at all pale or frightened or out of breath, Fred told me when I cross-examined him, though at the time he was too violently excited to note a detail of that sort. Indeed she smiled and spoke in an easy pleasant voice.

'Cramp,' she said, 'I have cramp.' Both the men were convinced of that.

Mr. Bunting was on the point of telling her to hold tight and she would be quite safe, when a little wave went almost entirely into his mouth and reduced him to wild splutterings.

'*We'll* get you in,' said Fred, or something of that sort, and so they all hung, bobbing in the water to the tune of Mr. Bunting's trouble. They seem to have rocked so for some time. Fred says the Sea Lady looked calm but a little puzzled and that she seemed to measure the distance shoreward. 'You *mean* to save me?' she asked him.

He was trying to think what could be done before his father drowned. 'We're saving you now,' he said.

'You'll take me ashore?'

As she seemed so cool he thought he would explain his plan of operations,

'Trying to get – end of ladder – kick with my legs. Only a few yards out of our depth – if we could only –'

'Minute-get my breath-moufu' sea-water,' said Mr. Bunting. *Splash!* wuff! . . .

And then it seemed to Fred that a little miracle happened. There was a swirl of the water like the swirl about a screw propeller, and he gripped the Sea Lady and the ladder just in time, as it seemed to him, to prevent his being washed far out into the Channel. His father vanished from his sight with an expression of astonishment just forming on his face and reappeared beside him, so far as back and legs are concerned, holding on to the ladder with a sort of death grip. And then behold! They had shifted a dozen yards inshore, and they were in less than five feet of water and Fred could feel the ground.

At its touch his amazement and dismay immediately gave way to the purest heroism. He thrust ladder and Sea Lady before him, abandoned the ladder and his now quite disordered parent, caught her tightly in his arms, and bore her up out of the water. The young ladies cried 'Saved!' the maids cried 'Saved!' Distant voices echoed 'Saved, Hooray!'

'I had cramp,' said the Sea Lady, with her lips against Fred's cheek and one eye on Mrs. Bunting. 'I am sure it was cramp . . . I've got it still.'

'I don't see anybody—' began Mrs. Bunting.

'Please carry me in,' said the Sea Lady, closing her eyes as if she were ill—though her cheek was flushed and warm. 'Carry me in.'

'Where?' gasped Fred.

'Carry me into the house,' she whispered to him.

'Which house?'

Mrs. Bunting came nearer.

'*Your* house,' said the Sea Lady, and shut her eyes for good and became oblivious to all further remarks.

'She— But I don't understand—' said Mrs. Bunting, addressing everybody . . .

And then it was they saw it. Nettie, the younger Miss Bunting, saw it first. She pointed, she says, before she could find words to speak. Then they all saw it! Miss Glendower, I believe, was the person who was last to see it. At any rate it would have been like her if she had been.

'Mother,' said Nettie, giving words to the general horror. '*Mother! She has a tail!*' And then the three maids and Mabel Glendower screamed one after the other.

'Look!' they cried. 'A tail!'

'Of all—' said Mrs. Bunting, and words failed her.

'*Oh!*' said Miss Glendower, and put her hand to her heart. And then one of the maids gave it a name.

'It's a mermaid!' screamed the maid, and then everyone screamed, 'It's a mermaid.'

MERMAID TALES CAN BE FOUND all over the world, and in some cultures women are seen as particularly adept at deep sea diving, such as Japan's 'sea women' or Ama. Writer Nina Mingya Powles, something of a mermaid herself – since first learning to swim in her local childhood pool in Borneo – elegantly explores their presence in stories from Japan, New Zealand, Indonesia and China.

'Pania is a young sea maiden who swims with sea creatures.'
Small Bodies of Water by Nina Mingya Powles[38]

The pond seems to contain layers of translucent pearls and blue-green clouds. A family of black tufted ducks floats around me as I become aware of what my body looks like: disappearing, half-swallowed by the deep. Here, there's nothing to push myself off from. I can't touch the bottom, I can't see more than a few inches ahead of me underwater. I am not sure where the shape of me ends and the dark water begins. The only sure thing is my body. I hold my breath and swim out towards the place where the sun touches the surface . . .

When I grew older I looked beyond the canon of Western mythology for myths of women who are neither human nor fish, but both. In Malaysia and Indonesia, dugongs – a type of marine mammal similar to manatees, both of the order Sirenia – are linked in traditional myth to half-fish half-human creatures. In ancient Chinese texts there are mentions of various kinds of mermaids, including a sea-dwelling people who weave silk from the fine filaments that hold molluscs onto rocks. In Japanese folklore, there is a fish creature with a human head called Ningyo. And we can be eager to attach the mythical status of 'mermaid' to the real world. Ama – sea women – come from generations of skin divers in Japan. They once dived for pearls with only their skins to protect them from cold waters; now they dive for shellfish while wearing traditional white hooded suits thought to ward off evil. On Jeju Island in South Korea, the Haenyeo women also make a living from free diving. Articles often evoke the women as figures from a forgotten past. 'The Last Mermaids of Japan', 'Haenyeo: The Elderly Mermaids of Jeju Island', 'Inside the Island of Sea Women' . . .

In the Māori myth Pania of the Reef, Pania is a young sea maiden who swims with sea creatures during the day and rests on land at night. One day she falls in love with a human Karitoki, who doesn't understand why she has to return to the sea each day. He consults a kaumatua, an elder, who tells him Pania won't be able to return to the sea as long as she eats food cooked by humans. Karitoki tricks her by putting a piece of food in her mouth while she sleeps. Pania wakes just in time and flees back to the sea, never to return again.

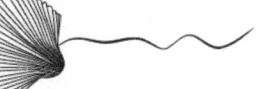

FEMINIST ANTHROPOLOGIST ELAINE MORGAN'S 1972 classic *The Descent of Woman* contains a feminist take on the idea of mermaids, arguing that women became semi-aquatic apes and then men followed them into the water.

This polemic – whether you believe in its central thesis or not – is a counterpoint to the way anthropological theories of the time typically centred on a male point of view: 'this is where we found the spears so this must be the men's area' or 'women developed breasts because men found them attractive' (no joke; that is a real theory).

Morgan theorises that those human ancestors who came down from the trees were easy meat for predators and so died out – except for those on the coast and rivers who took to beach life, slipping in and out of the water. It was the women who led the way, escaping from both predators and men.

Over millennia, Morgan argues, women developed large buttocks for sitting reasonably comfortably on the pebbly beach, their genitals moved round to the front for protection from sharp stones and gritty sand, and they grew long hair on their heads for babies to cling onto as they foraged and swam in the shallows.

Women also developed a human nose, with the nostrils protected by cartilage unlike in monkeys, making it easier to hold their breath underwater. People, Morgan theorises, started to enjoy swimming once they covered their nostrils. The only other monkey with a nose a bit like a human's – the splashy, doggy-paddling pro, the proboscis monkey – also 'delights in swimming'.

'With piercing squeals of terror she ran straight into the sea.'
The Descent of Woman by Elaine Morgan[39]

Hundreds of miles away [from the overheating interior] near the coast lived a female cousin of the same species, another timid, hairy, undifferentiated Miocene-type ape. Her piece of forest was shrinking, too. As the heat and the dryness spread out from the baking heart of Africa, it became reduced to a narrowing strip; the larger and fiercer arboreans drove her away, just as her cousin had been driven, from poaching on their dwindling preserves. She also couldn't digest grass; she also had a greedy and hectoring mate; she also lacked fighting canine teeth; she also was hampered by a clinging infant; and she also was chased by a carnivore and found there was no tree she could run up to escape. However, in front of her there was a large sheet of water. With piercing squeals of terror she ran straight into the sea. The carnivore was a species of cat and didn't like wetting his feet; and moreover, though he had twice her body weight, she was accustomed like most tree-dwellers to adopting an upright posture, even though she used four legs for locomotion. She was thus able to go farther into the water than he could without drowning. She went right in up to her neck and waited there . . .

Whenever anything alarming happened on the landward side – or sometimes just because it was getting so hot – she would go back into the water, up to her waist, or even up to her neck. This meant, of course, that she had to walk upright on her two hind legs. It was slow and ungainly, especially at first, but it was absolutely essential if she wanted to keep her head above water. She isn't the only creature who has ever had to learn to do it. Although, as we have seen, she is almost unique in having learned to walk upright all the time, there is another mammal who does it for part of the time, and probably for the same reason. The beaver, whose ancestors also spent a good deal of time in shallow water, whenever she transporting building materials or carrying her baby around, has the habit of getting up on her hind legs and proceeding by means of a perfectly serviceable bipedal gait.

She was very relieved to notice that even the large alarming-looking things that sometimes clambered out of the sea – things like seals, and giant turtles, and various kinds of sea cow – which were much commoner in those days – all proved to be very slow and clumsy and helpless on land, and in most cases totally disinclined to fight back when attacked . . .

She spent so much time in the water that her fur became nothing but a nuisance to her. Oftener than not, mammals who return to the water and stay there long enough, especially in warm climates, lose their hair as a perfectly natural consequence. Wet fur on land is no use to anyone, and fur in the water tends to slow down your swimming. She began to turn into a naked ape for the same reason as the porpoise turned into a naked cetacean, the hippopotamus into a naked ungulate, the walrus into a naked pinniped, and the manatee into a naked sirenian. As her fur began to disappear she felt more and more comfortable in the water, and that is where she spent the Pliocene, patiently waiting for conditions in the interior to improve. I believe these are the 'circumstances special to the point of disbelief' which explain how an anthropoid began to turn into a hominid.

Morgan also had a real-life origin story for the mermaid legends – she posited that they could have been inspired by the dugong, commonly known as the sea cow, which grazes on sea grass in the shallow coastal waters of the Indian and western Pacific oceans.

Face to face for aquatics is so consistent a rule that they don't even have to be marine to resort to it – it holds good for freshwater divers also. The actual mating of beavers is not often seen, but it has been observed on Russian beaver farms, and, as Lars Wilsson relates it: 'The scent of the female in heat is presumably enough to make the male sufficiently sensually stimulated, and when she goes into the water in a particular way he follows, and mating takes place stomach to stomach, the animals swimming slowly forward.'

And to return to the sirenians, a report on the dugong by H. A. E. Goohar confirms that these tropical sea cows fit into the face-to-face aquatic pattern. The same report offers the most probable solution to the mystery of the mariner and the mermaid. It points out that there is a striking resemblance between the genitalia of dugongs and those of human beings: and that in the Red Sea area there is an oral tradition that in former centuries a sailor after months at sea who found a dugong in the shallows – large, docile, warm-blooded, air-breathing, smooth-skinned, female-breasted, and with ventral genital organs which remarkably well fitted his own wouldn't worry overmuch if she was comparatively faceless. In those days such a sea maiden may well have represented temptation even though she has never learned to sing a siren's song.

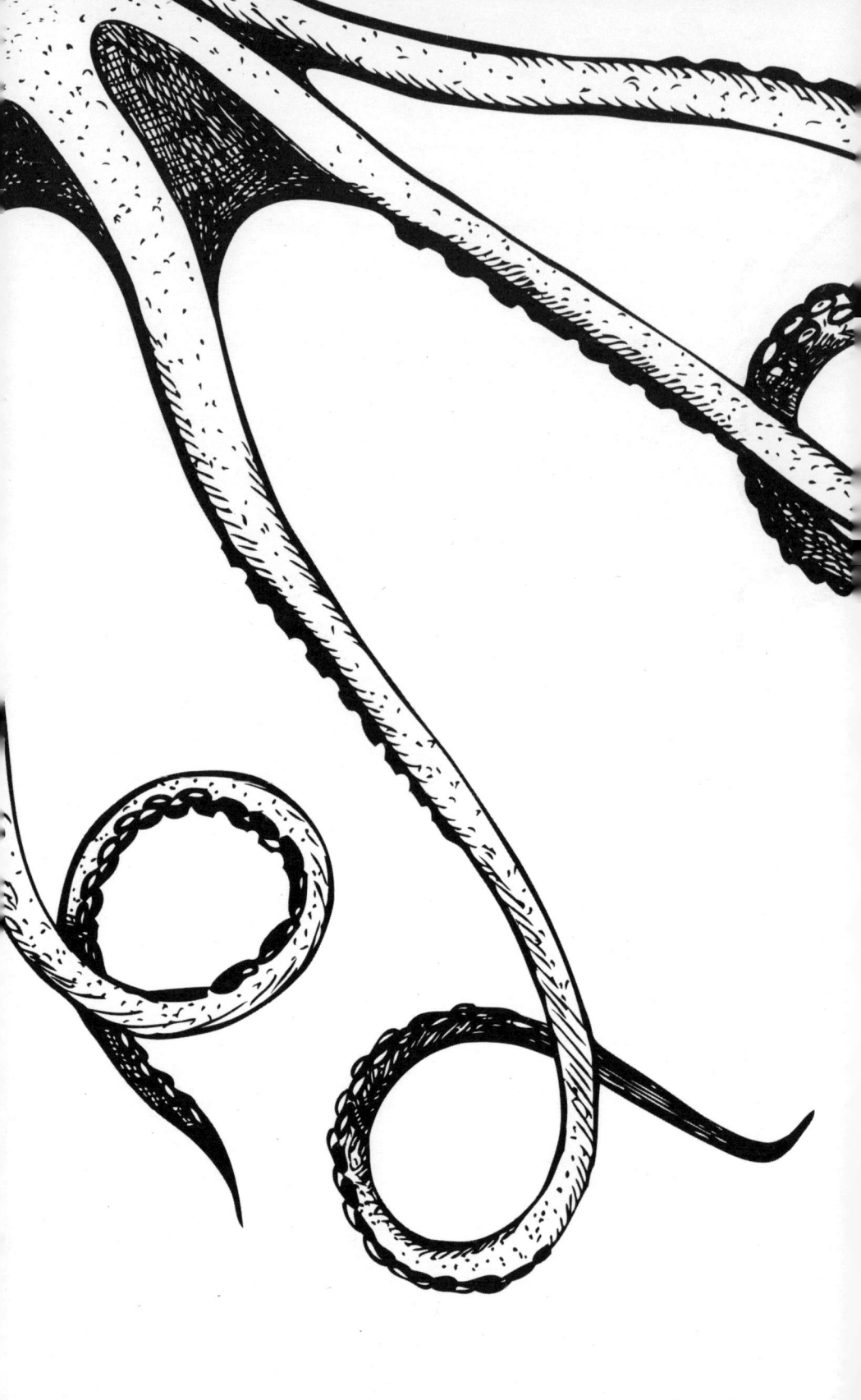

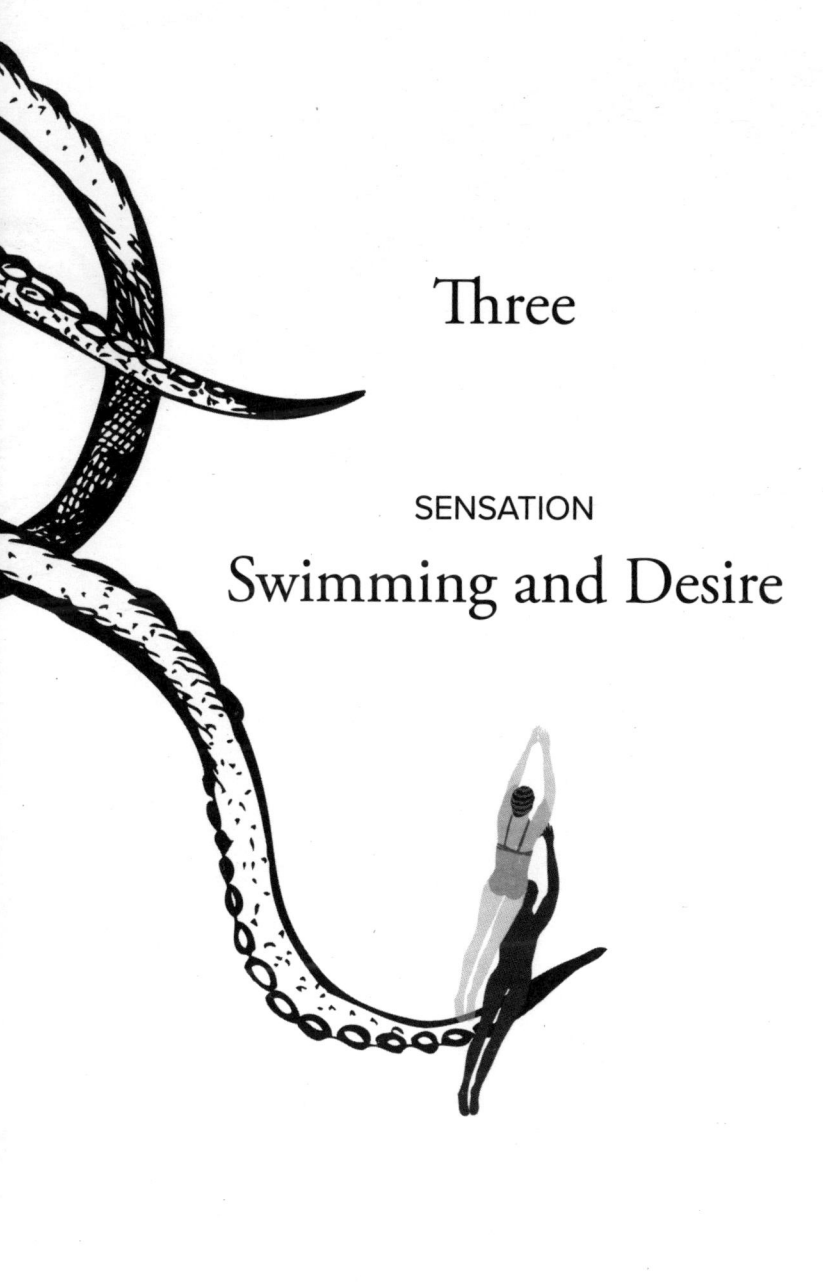

Three

SENSATION

Swimming and Desire

THE FEEL OF THE WATER tingling against bare skin can be a sensuous experience – and the longing for it sharp. In 'Innisfree', the poet W. B. Yeats wrote about carrying a 'bee-loud glade' in his heart 'as he stands on the pavement or on the roadways grey'. Many wild swimmers pounding city streets console themselves with an inner, heart-held picture of themselves battling – energetically battling – the waves.

Then there is contact with others – swimming involves removing the outer layer and revealing the body. When we swim, the water connects us, but also keeps us apart, presenting a challenge even to a simple kiss. It can be a space of flirtation, of foreplay, of building desire. 'No petting' was the iconic rule on swimming pool walls. That and a 'No smoking' cartoon of a louche dude blowing three perfect smoke rings before taking a dip.

CHAPTER I

Feeling Water

DURING THE PANDEMIC, I WAS in the Highlands and starting to think about taking up wild swimming, but a bit daunted by the freezing water. My daughter passed on a link to ice swimmer Gilly McArthur's podcasts, which I found really helpful, particularly in their suggestion never to mention the 'c-word' (cold). Gilly's advice was to work up to swimming and not to rush it or force yourself to enter the water, and the first few times I ventured to the shores of the shallow lochan near our house, I only paddled and tried to simply absorb the sensation without, as they say, judgement.

'The icy water is now at my waist. I take a deep breath.'
'Where Ice Meets Fluidity', from *Taking the Plunge* by Vicky Allan and Anna Deacon[40]

Gilly McArthur

I feel heightened like someone has turned the volume dial up on all my senses. The cool wind meets my ears, now from the north-west; it's biting, whispering and brushing my face and arms. High up a buzzard cries on a peak in the clouds. My heart beats in my throat and then I feel it down to my warm fingertips. My skin hums, a familiar, welcome sensation. It starts in the base of my spine, saunters up my back to the top of my head, and I feel a wave of calm. I breathe deeply, setting my mind, taking that first step.

Cracking with a sound like small twigs snapping, the ice on the shoreline is thin and slippery in places. Placing a definite foot between icy glassy shards and slick, cold rock, I feel the first touch of water. Now I'm connected to this element of water. This heady, visceral moment. I gently push the ice I have cut out of the way as I wade in, aware of its danger. I sense its weight; yet I'm amazed too at its hefty mass as it floats so easily. It's sharp, about an inch or so thick, and milky white. The sounds it makes, dull clinks of glass, and bubbles forming under the ice sheet where my disruption is now sending fresh air under the thick skin of the tarn.

The icy water is now at my waist. I take a deep breath in, and out, and then let go. Breathing out fully to break from my conscious reaction to the cold; pushing against my instinct to breathe in. I focus on my hands moving through the inky peaty water, pushing the ice from my path and, crucially, my neck as I swim. Today the water feels clean, smooth, silky. It can be dense, heavy and prickly, but not today. That's the magic of swimming in ice.

And now I'm swimming. Intentional strokes, my whole body moving, floating through the tarn. Sight engaging where solid ice meets fluidity. There is no judgement here – judgement leads to creeping fear – so it's little more than a gentle awareness of my surroundings. Holding everything as lightly as water flow itself. Observing without judgement these wild sensations of cold. I'm smiling, though, so I know this is wonderful, comforting, effortless.

After a while my limbs feel heavier. It begins under my biceps; then my toes start to feel different, right at the tips. I always make sure I have far more time than I need, so I turn and head for shore for the last time, to get out and get dry and get warm. I'll be back, probably tomorrow, to this deep profound connection to now. Moment upon moment of bliss, joy and calm. My liquid meditation.

BUT STILL, THE COLD IS an undeniable part of the experience and the sudden obliteration it brings is an irresistible draw to many. The feeling of being overwhelmed by the cold is one that was captured by the Cairngorms writer, Nan Shepherd, in her influential book, *The Living Mountain*, when she describes a plunge into a mountain pool.

'The whole skin has this delightful sensitivity.'
The Living Mountain by Nan Shepherd[41]

In fording a swollen stream, one's strongest sensation is of the pouring strength of the water against one's limbs, the effort to poise the body against it gives significance to this simple act of walking through running water. Early in the season the water may be so cold that one has no sensation except of cold; the whole being retracts itself, uses all its resources to endure this icy delight. But in the heat the freshness of the water slides over the skin like shadow. The whole skin has this delightful sensitivity; it feels the sun, it feels the wind running inside one's garment, it feels water closing on it as one slips under – the catch in the breath, like a wave held back, the glow that releases one's entire cosmos, running to the ends of the body as the spent wave runs out upon the sand. This plunge into the cold water of a mountain pool seems for a brief moment to disintegrate the very self; it is not to be borne: one is lost: stricken: annihilated. Then life pours back.

IN THE CLASSIC POETRY COLLECTION of the mid-nineteenth century, *Leaves of Grass*, the book that changed poetry for ever by abandoning metre and rhyme, Walt Whitman imagines the sea as a lover beckoning him to bathe.

'An unseen hand also pass'd over their bodies.'
'Song of Myself' by Walt Whitman[42]

> You sea! I resign myself to you also—I guess what you mean,
> I behold from the beach your crooked inviting fingers,
> I believe you refuse to go back without feeling of me,
> We must have a turn together, I undress, hurry me out of sight of
>   the land,
> Cushion me soft, rock me in billowy drowse,
> Dash me with amorous wet, I can repay you.
> Sea of stretch'd ground-swells,
> Sea breathing broad and convulsive breaths,
> Sea of the brine of life and of unshovell'd yet always-ready graves,
> Howler and scooper of storms, capricious and dainty sea,
> I am integral with you, I too am of one phase and of all phases.

EMILY DICKINSON, A CONTEMPORARY OF Whitman's, was little known during her lifetime but later came to be regarded as one of the giants of American poetry. This poem is ostensibly a poem about being overwhelmed by the tide. It is generally read as a metaphor for lust or sexual awakening, with the sea standing in for a lover's touch.

'But no Man moved Me – till the Tide.'
'I started Early – Took my Dog' by Emily Dickinson[43]

I started Early – Took my Dog –
And visited the Sea –
The Mermaids in the Basement
Came out to look at me –

And Frigates – in the Upper Floor
Extended Hempen Hands –
Presuming Me to be a Mouse –
Aground – opon the Sands –

But no Man moved Me – till the Tide
Went past my simple Shoe –
And past my Apron – and my Belt
And past my Boddice – too –

And made as He would eat me up –
As wholly as a Dew
Opon a Dandelion's Sleeve –
And then – I started – too –

And He – He followed – close behind –
I felt His Silver Heel
Opon my Ancle – Then My Shoes
Would overflow with Pearl –

Until We met the Solid Town –
No One He seemed to know –

And bowing – with a Mighty look –
At me – The Sea withdrew –

~

THE FRENCH DIARIST PAUL VALÉRY called swimming 'fornication avec l'onde'.

'The body spreads itself, draws itself in, understands itself.'
'On Swimming', in *Mediterranean Inspiration* by Paul Valéry[44]

I seem to rediscover and know myself again when I return to the water. To plunge into the mass and the movement, to be active from head to toe, to roll in that pure and deep element, breathe in and breathe out the divine saltness—this for me is nearest to the act of love, the activity in which my body becomes all signs and all powers, as a hand opens and closes, speaks and acts.

Here all the body spreads itself, draws itself in, understands itself, spends itself trying to exhaust all its possibilities. It touches her, wishes to seize her, embrace her; it goes mad with life and its own freedom of movement; it loves her, possesses her, with her it engenders a thousand strange ideas. Through her, I am the man I wish to be. My body becomes the immediate instrument of my mind, and yet the author of all its ideas. All is clarified for me. I understand to the full what love might be.

CHAPTER II

Erotic Encounters

WRITERS OFTEN RETURN TO THE entanglement between water and sexual attraction in passages about erotic love. In *The Sharing Economy* by my dear friend Sophie Berrebi, Gabrielle, a forty-something mother in an open marriage, begins dating over what is called 'the app'. It's a radical tale of sexual awakening, but also a journey through art, philosophy, the impact of a new technology and the city of Amsterdam. At one point, a lover takes Gabrielle for a date to a swimming lake near Abcoude, south of the city.

'Come, let's swim!'
The Sharing Economy by Sophie Berrebi[45]

Emil began undressing on the boat, causing it to sway perilously from side to side. I did not have swimming things with me; besides; the water would be freezing.

He brushed my excuses away: 'I brought some towels; but I did not want you to know anything about where we were going. We are completely alone here; we can swim naked.'

Emil had shed his clothes entirely and stood on the boat, his slim freckled body and rust-coloured hair contrasting against the matching blues of sky and water.

'Come!' He climbed out of the boat and splashed into the water.

Jumping ship sounded like a particularly bad idea to· me. The possibilities of getting a heart attack from the cold water, the boat that might drift away, the sea-creatures that were bound to be lurking around waiting for us as a treat. Emil laughed. I really was a city girl.

I removed my t-shirt and long skirt, and stretched on the boat letting the sun touch the exposed flesh. I slowly peeled off my underwear. Emil swam further into the lake. I slowly, clumsily clambered out, sensing the hard edge of the boat catching and cutting into my thighs as I flipped my weight and eased myself slowly into the cool water. I felt the cold liquid lick my body and gasped as it trickled between my thighs. I slid further, lowered my hips into the cold water. I let go from the boat and let out an involuntary scream as the tip of my feet touched the soft, muddy bottom of the water. I had never swum in fresh water before. Emil came back towards the boat and we swam out together, keeping our bodies as parallel to the surface as we could to bathe in the warmer patches of water. All around us the strong rays of sun pierced through the lake's trembling surface, creating light tunnels that tunnelled into its depths. Further away the rays of the sun bounced off the surface causing it to sparkle and shimmer, and the dense bushes of reeds on the banks took on an even brighter green.

We clambered back onto the small boat after a while and rowed over to a short strip of land nearby, a miniature peninsula where we finished drying off and laid on the grass, I felt the sun slowly erase the cold off my limbs, and shroud them in a comfortable warmth. I gazed at the infinite cloudless sky as Emil nuzzled my neck and wrapped his body around mine. We lay still.

A few ducks surrounded the boat, a heron stood on a grassy bank across a narrower stretch of water. We walked around the strip of land, naked. I asked Emil to tell me the names of the plants in the water around us.

'Water soldiers': he pointed at the green spikes emerging from the surface, in the shape of a crown. 'And these yellow flowers here, bladder-worts, they are carnivorous plants.' Small insects buzzed around; the rough grasses tickled my feet.

We spent the rest of the afternoon rowing across the lake, passing through waterways small and wide, dipping into the water, kissing and fondling on the grass, looking at the small white waterlilies unfolding their leaves on the quiet surface of the pool. We never saw another boat. The light became bluer as we feasted on tins of smoky mackerel and sardines, dunking chunks of bread in the oil, and a few apples and cherries, which we washed down with sparkling water.

SOPHIE'S BOOK DESCRIBES A WAY of living – an open marriage – that is not entirely new. There are echoes of this in D. H. Lawrence's relationship with his wife Frieda. She was from a very different background from the miner's son and had little time for bourgeois British notions of propriety.

Frieda grew up on the fringes of the Imperial German court in the late nineteenth century and was related to the First World War flying ace known as 'the Red Baron'. Familiar with the work of Freud, at a time when this was unusual, Frieda was able to introduce Lawrence to some of his ideas. Frieda, who left her first marriage and children to be with the man she knew as Bert, believed that 'if only love were free' it would make for a happier world.

Bert, while not openly gay, appeared to struggle with his feelings for other men in an age when homosexuality was often suppressed; it remained illegal for over thirty years after his death. The Lawrences' relationship became strained in later years. A friend wrote that when they swam together at hot springs she often saw 'great black and blue bruises on Frieda's blonde flesh'. American poet Witter Bynner, who travelled with the couple in South America, observed Bert being abusive and controlling with Frieda, including insisting that she dress modestly for swimming, in calico bloomers.

But Frieda seems to have regularly escaped the marriage for her own erotic adventures. The couple's neighbour, the Scottish composer Cecil Gray, hinted at an affair with Frieda and wrote that he did not think that Bert and Frieda had a sexual relationship by that time. Nor was this Frieda's only affair. There is this wonderful story, from David Garnett's memoirs, telling of how Frieda once swam naked across a river to make love to a woodcutter. Bert drew on Frieda for many of the female characters in his fiction – although they were never quite as free-spirited as she.

'Farewell philosopher! I love a peasant.'
'Frieda and Lawrence' by David Garnett, in *D. H. Lawrence: Novelist, Poet, Prophet* (edited by Stephen Spender)[46]

I was a science student aged twenty and was spending part of the long vacation in Munich. My father wrote suggesting I should see Lawrence who invited me to Icking where he had taken a room. Frieda was then living in the neighbouring village of Wolfratshausen in a cottage belonging either to Jaffe or her elder sister. It was a very hot day and when the little train had decanted me and a crowd of perspiring Bavarians, there was no difficulty in my recognising Lawrence or he, me.

He was a slightly built, narrow-chested man, thin and tall with mud-coloured hair, a small moustache and a hairpin chin. He was obviously British working class. It was his eyes that charmed you and in two minutes I had fallen under their spell. They were full of gaiety, of an unspoken promise: 'We'll have fun together!' That unspoken promise was not broken. We did have fun. Lawrence was at that period – perhaps always – more alive than most human beings.

We went back to his room and he soon suggested that we walk through the woods to Wolfratshausen. We found Frieda lying in a hammock. She gave a lazy roll and a leap and was standing up, greeting me. There was something in her powerful face, with its straight nose, in her gold-green eyes and her movements, which made me think of a lioness. Frieda was a noble and splendid animal. I could see at once that she was free and truthful and honest. She was not a bitch – though she did some things that would have led some men to call her one.

I found out that summer – Lawrence must have told me – that after they had had a row, she had gone down to the Isar and swum over to where a woodcutter was working, had made love with him and had swum back – just to show Lawrence that she was free to do what she liked. I told the story to Anna Wickham who wrote a poem about it. I quote it here because I like it . . . I don't suppose she ever showed it to them after they had become friends three years later . . .

My love shall be a sphere of silence and of light
Where love is all alone with love's delight
Here is a woodcutter who is so weak
With love of me he cannot speak.
Tell me dumb man, am I pleasant, am I pleasant?
Farewell philosopher! I love a peasant.

~~~

IN THIS PASSAGE FROM D. H. LAWRENCE'S *Women in Love*, published in 1920, the character Gudrun is excited by seeing the naked Gerald Crich leap into the lake – the inappropriately named Willey Water. Gudrun rails against social constraints, without actually throwing them aside.

'"How I envy him," she said, in low, desirous tones.'
Women in Love by D. H. Lawrence[47]

When Gudrun and Ursula came to Willey Water, the lake lay all grey and visionary, stretching into the moist, translucent vista of trees and meadow. Fine electric activity in sound came from the dumbles below the road, the birds piping one against the other, and water mysteriously plashing, issuing from the lake. The two girls drifted swiftly along. In front of them, at the corner of the lake, near the road, was a mossy boat-house under a walnut tree, and a little landing-stage where a boat was moored, wavering like a shadow on the still grey water, below the green, decayed poles. All was shadowy with coming summer.

Suddenly, from the boat-house, a white figure ran out, frightening in its swift sharp transit, across the old landing-stage. It launched in a white arc through the air, there was a bursting of the water, and among the smooth ripples a swimmer was making out to space, in a centre of faintly heaving motion. The whole otherworld, wet and remote, he had to himself. He could move into the pure translucency of the grey, uncreated water.

Gudrun stood by the stone wall, watching.

'How I envy him,' she said, in low, desirous tones.

'Ugh!' shivered Ursula. 'So cold!'

'Yes, but how good, how really fine, to swim out there!' The sisters stood watching the swimmer move further into the grey, moist, full space of the water, pulsing with his own small, invading motion, and arched over with mist and dim woods.

'Don't you wish it were you?' asked Gudrun, looking at Ursula.

'I do,' said Ursula. 'But I'm not sure—it's so wet.'

'No,' said Gudrun, reluctantly. She stood watching the motion on the bosom of the water, as if fascinated. He, having swum a certain distance, turned round and was swimming on his back, looking along the water at the two girls by the wall. In the faint wash of motion, they could see his ruddy face, and could feel him watching them.

'It is Gerald Crich,' said Ursula.

'I know,' replied Gudrun.

And she stood motionless gazing over the water at the face which washed up and down on the flood, as he swam steadily. From his separate element he saw them and he exulted to himself because of his own advantage, his possession of a world to himself. He was immune and perfect. He loved his own vigorous, thrusting motion, and the violent impulse of the very cold water against his limbs, buoying him up. He could see the girls watching him a way off, outside, and that pleased him. He lifted his arm from the water, in a sign to them.

'He is waving,' said Ursula.

'Yes,' replied Gudrun. They watched him. He waved again, with a strange movement of recognition across the difference.

'Like a Nibelung,' laughed Ursula. Gudrun said nothing, only stood still looking over the water.

Gerald suddenly turned, and was swimming away swiftly, with a side stroke. He was alone now, alone and immune in the middle of the waters, which he had all to himself. He exulted in his isolation in the new element, unquestioned and unconditioned. He was happy, thrusting with his legs and all his body, without bond or connection anywhere, just himself in the watery world.

Gudrun envied him almost painfully. Even this momentary possession of pure isolation and fluidity seemed to her so terribly desirable that she felt herself as if damned, out there on the high-road.

'God, what it is to be a man!' she cried.

'What?' exclaimed Ursula in surprise.

'The freedom, the liberty, the mobility!' cried Gudrun, strangely flushed and brilliant. 'You're a man, you want to do a thing, you do it. You haven't the thousand obstacles a woman has in front of her.'

Ursula wondered what was in Gudrun's mind, to occasion this outburst. She could not understand.

'What do you want to do?' she asked.

'Nothing,' cried Gudrun, in swift refutation. 'But supposing I did. Supposing I want to swim up that water. It is impossible, it is one of the impossibilities of life, for me to take my clothes off now and jump in. But isn't it ridiculous, doesn't it simply prevent our living!' She was so hot, so flushed, so furious, that Ursula was puzzled.

~

FOR EDNA PONTELLIER, IN KATE CHOPIN'S 1899 proto-feminist novella, *The Awakening*, the sea and nature are a realm of sensuality, and her connection to them is part of her awakening. It is a space apart from the constrictions and expectations that society places on a woman. The book is set on the Louisiana Gulf Coast, where Edna, a 24-year-old Creole mother, is spending the summer. Her much older husband comes and goes from the house, controlling and undermining her. The sea is key to Edna's awakening. It is the stimulant.

Towards the end of this powerful, short book, she enters its waters for a last swim, and it is suggested that she drowns. When published, the book was met with scandalised reviews, criticising the immorality of Edna's rebellion against social norms. But for Chopin, who had been advised to write by her doctor and friend as therapy for depression, writing the novel was indeed a lifesaver. By the time of her death a few years later of a stroke, Chopin had achieved recognition as a local author in her home town of St Louis.

In this excerpt, Edna bathes with a young man, Robert LeBrun. These episodes, never properly described but sometimes referred to as 'adventures out on the water', take on a note of charged erotic mystery. From the first chapter we sense that something, perhaps still nascent, is going on between Edna and Robert. Her husband, Léonce Pontellier, observes them returning from the sea, and remarks, 'What folly! to bathe at such an hour in such heat!'

Robert is described as a serial 'devoted attendant' of young women. One afternoon after he has watched her paint, leaning his head on her arm, he asks, 'Are you bathing?' They walk down to sea together. What happens there, again, is not fully described, but the following passage hints at the attraction between them, as well as the sensuous draw of the sea – itself a metaphor for some kind of sexual awakening.

'The voice of the sea is seductive; never ceasing, whispering, clamoring, murmuring.'
The Awakening by Kate Chopin[48]

Edna Pontellier could not have told why, wishing to go to the beach with Robert, she should in the first place have declined, and in the second place have followed in obedience to one of the two contradictory impulses which impelled her.

A certain light was beginning to dawn dimly within her,—the light which, showing the way, forbids it.

At that early period it served but to bewilder her. It moved her to dreams, to thoughtfulness, to the shadowy anguish which had overcome her the midnight when she had abandoned herself to tears.

In short, Mrs. Pontellier was beginning to realize her position in the universe as a human being, and to recognize her relations as an individual to the world within and about her. This may seem like a ponderous weight of wisdom to descend upon the soul of a young woman of twenty-eight—perhaps more wisdom than the Holy Ghost is usually pleased to vouchsafe to any woman.

But the beginning of things, of a world especially, is necessarily vague, tangled, chaotic, and exceedingly disturbing. How few of us ever emerge from such beginning! How many souls perish in its tumult!

The voice of the sea is seductive; never ceasing, whispering, clamoring, murmuring, inviting the soul to wander for a spell in abysses of solitude; to lose itself in mazes of inward contemplation.

The voice of the sea speaks to the soul. The touch of the sea is sensuous, enfolding the body in its soft, close embrace.

On another occasion, Robert suggests that a group of the vacationers go for a mystic bathe under a mystic moon.

At all events Robert proposed it, and there was not a dissenting voice. There was not one but was ready to follow when he led the way. He did not lead the way, however, he directed the way; and he himself loitered behind with the lovers, who had betrayed a disposition to linger and hold themselves apart. He walked between them, whether with malicious or mischievous intent was not wholly clear, even to himself.

The Pontelliers and Ratignolles walked ahead; the women leaning upon the arms of their husbands. Edna could hear Robert's voice behind them, and could sometimes hear what he said. She wondered why he did not join them. It was unlike him not to. Of late he had sometimes held away from her for an entire day, redoubling his devotion upon the next and the next, as though to make up for hours that had been lost. She missed him the days when some pretext served to take him away from her, just as one misses the sun on a cloudy day without having thought much about the sun when it was shining.

The people walked in little groups toward the beach. They talked and laughed; some of them sang. There was a band playing down at Klein's hotel, and the strains reached them faintly, tempered by the distance. There were strange, rare odors abroad—a tangle of the sea smell and of weeds and damp, new-plowed earth, mingled with the heavy perfume of a field of white blossoms somewhere near. But the night sat lightly upon the sea and the land. There was no weight of darkness; there were no shadows. The white light of the moon had fallen upon the world like the mystery and the softness of sleep.

Most of them walked into the water as though into a native element. The sea was quiet now, and swelled lazily in broad billows that melted into one another and did not break except upon the beach in little foamy crests that coiled back like slow, white serpents.

Edna had attempted all summer to learn to swim. She had received instructions from both the men and women; in some instances from the children. Robert had pursued a system of lessons almost daily; and he was nearly at the point of discouragement in realizing the futility of his efforts. A certain ungovernable dread hung about her when in the water, unless there was a hand near by that might reach out and reassure her.

But that night she was like the little tottering, stumbling, clutching child, who of a sudden realizes its powers, and walks for the first time alone, boldly and with over-confidence. She could have shouted for joy. She did shout for joy, as with a sweeping stroke or two she lifted her body to the surface of the water.

A feeling of exultation overtook her, as if some power of significant import had been given her to control the working of her body and her soul. She grew daring and reckless, overestimating her strength. She wanted to swim far out, where no woman had swum before.

Her unlooked-for achievement was the subject of wonder, applause, and admiration. Each one congratulated himself that his special teachings had accomplished this desired end.

'How easy it is!' she thought. 'It is nothing,' she said aloud; 'why did I not discover before that it was nothing. Think of the time I have lost splashing about like a baby!' She would not join the groups in their sports and bouts, but intoxicated with her newly conquered power, she swam out alone.

She turned her face seaward to gather in an impression of space and solitude, which the vast expanse of water, meeting and melting with the moonlit sky, conveyed to her excited fancy. As she swam she seemed to be reaching out for the unlimited in which to lose herself.

Following the swim, Edna and Robert walk back to her house together and he assists her into a hammock. The sexual tension is undeniable.

He seated himself again and rolled a cigarette, which he smoked in silence. Neither did Mrs. Pontellier speak. No multitude of words could have been more significant than those moments of silence, or more pregnant with the first-felt throbbings of desire.

When the voices of the bathers were heard approaching, Robert said good-night. She did not answer him. He thought she was asleep. Again she watched his figure pass in and out of the strips of moonlight as he walked away.

~

OSCAR WILDE'S PROLONGED EROTIC POEM 'Charmides' caused a scandal in strait-laced late-Victorian Britain. The mother of a friend cut it out – literally, with scissors – of a book of Wilde's called *Poems* and let it be known that the celebrated wit would no longer be welcome in her home.

The story is about a beautiful Greek boy who falls in love with a statue of Athena and later leaps into the sea to be united with her. After he drowns, a nymph falls in love with his corpse. Here she broods over the lad's unconscious body, fantasising that he will awake and make love to her under the waves. The disturbing story and ornate style might not appeal to modern taste, but Wilde once said that this was his most finished and perfect poem.

'A blue wave will be our canopy.'
'Charmides' by Oscar Wilde[49]

She said, 'He will awake, I know him well,
He will awake at evening when the sun
Hangs his red shield on Corinth's citadel;
This sleep is but a cruel treachery
To make me love him more, and in some cavern of the sea

TAKE ME TO THE RIVER

'We two will sit upon a throne of pearl,
And a blue wave will be our canopy,
And at our feet the water-snakes will curl
In all their amethystine panoply
Of diamonded mail, and we will mark
The mullets swimming by the mast of some storm-foundered bark,

'And tremulous opal-hued anemones
Will wave their purple fringes where we tread
Upon the mirrored floor, and argosies
Of fishes flecked with tawny scales will thread
The drifting cordage of the shattered wreck,
And honey-coloured amber beads our twining limbs will deck.'

~~~

WALT WHITMAN'S 'SONG OF MYSELF' is quoted on page 128 on the subject of longing for the water. Later in the long poem, whose explicit sexual imagery was scandalous at the time, the narrator puts himself in the persona of a shy lady in a house by the river. She longingly watches twenty-eight naked young men who come to bathe there, before losing herself in congress with the twenty-ninth.

'Twenty-eight young men bathe by the shore.'
'Song of Myself' by Walt Whitman[50]

Twenty-eight young men bathe by the shore,
Twenty-eight young men and all so friendly;
Twenty-eight years of womanly life and all so lonesome.

She owns the fine house by the rise of the bank,
She hides handsome and richly drest aft the blinds of the window.
Which of the young men does she like the best?
Ah the homeliest of them is beautiful to her.
Where are you off to, lady? for I see you,
You splash in the water there, yet stay stock still in your room.
Dancing and laughing along the beach came the twenty-ninth bather,
The rest did not see her, but she saw them and loved them.
The beards of the young men glisten'd with wet, it ran from their long hair,
Little streams pass'd all over their bodies.
An unseen hand also pass'd over their bodies,
It descended tremblingly from their temples and ribs.
The young men float on their backs, their white bellies bulge to the sun,
they do not ask who seizes fast to them,
They do not know who puffs and declines with pendant and bending arch,
They do not think whom they souse with spray . . .

~~~~~~

IN ENGLISH NOVELIST ALAN HOLLINGHURST'S landmark literary sensation set in the early 1980s, there are frequent scenes set in the swimming pool at the narrator Will's club, the Corinthian, where he cruises for men in a steamily homoerotic atmosphere.

'I went to swim most days.'
The Swimming-Pool Library by Alan Hollinghurst[51]

The swimming-pool at the Corry is reached down a spiral staircase from the changing-rooms. It is the most subterranean zone of the Club, its high coffered ceiling supporting the floor of the gym above. Corinthian pillars at each corner are an allusion to ancient Rome, and you half expect to see the towel-girt figures of Charlton Heston and Tony Curtis deep in senatorial conspiracy. Instead, a bored attendant paces around the narrow mosaic border of the pool in flip-flops . . .

This makes the pool seem remote from the rest of the world, but the impression is lessened by the PA system which interrupts its continuous relay of music – insipid pop on weekdays, classical on Sundays – to call members to the phone or to reception. It is the camp voice of Michael that one normally hears, wringing the wildest insinuations out of words such as guest and occupant. Those who know his ways greet each announcement with a delight unshared by the novice; in my first week at the club the disdainful announcement that 'Mr Beckwith has a man in reception' had brought a round of silly laughter as I walked, blushing, from the gym. And the pool is a busy place. Except for certain mournful periods – early afternoons, Sunday evenings, there is a crowd: friends are racing, practised divers arch into the water making barely a splash, the agile avoid the slow, groups sit in a dripping line on the edge, feet flicking the water, cocks shrunken by the cold sticking up comically in their trunks.

Miles of serious swimming are wound up in those twenty-five yards each day, and though some dally between lengths, of most you see only the heave of breaststrokers' backs, the misted goggles and gasping, half-averted mouths of crawlers, the incessant cleaving movements of their arms, and the bubbling wakes of their feet.

I went to swim most days, sometimes after exercises on the mats in the gym or shortish turn in the weights room. It was a bizarre occupation, numbing and yet satisfying. I swam fast, alternating crawl and breaststroke, with a length of butterfly every ten. My mind would count its daily fifty lengths as automatically as a photocopier; and at the same time it would wander. Absorbed in thought I barely noticed the half-hour one unfaltering span of pure physical exercise – elapse.

This evening I thought of Arthur a lot, running real and projected conversations through my mind as I tumble-turned from length into length [before going up to the showers]. As I pushed open the swing door with its steamed-up little window designed, like those in restaurants, to prevent hurrying people from knocking each other flat, I heard the hiss of the crowded showers, and felt the warm, dense atmosphere of the place in my throat and on my skin. I sauntered along between the two files of hot jots whose spray danced up off the black tiles, shifting or suddenly cutting off as the men, naked or in their trunks, edged about, soaped a foot raised against the wall, gave their stomachs resounding smacks, or turned, as the doors to the outside world thwacked open, to see what beauty had arrived. Exchanging short greetings with a couple of chaps I scarcely knew, I chose a vacant position between a pale, ravaged-looking youth with tattoos snaking up his arms and a huge dark brown man, six foot eight tall at a guess, very round and heavy, with an enormous childish face and not a hair on his head – or, I soon found, anywhere on his body. His sleek, heavy cock, cushioned on a tight, crinkled scrotum, stuck out from beneath a roll of fat. He was soaping himself vigorously, leaving a silky smear over his smooth, plump expanses of back and belly: and with cheery unselfconsciousness singing as he went about it. I nodded to him, as if to say that I could see he was happy enough, then, and he grinned back in way that suggested a fond, exuberant disposition. I felt that he might stroke me as a golem does some little girl who trusts him, or inadvertently crush me to death. I set down my soap box and shampoo, let the water drum on my shoulders, and looked about.

At the Corry the men undress at their lockers, and then bring their towels to the duckboarded place at the end of the shower room. Often those who have swum still have their trunks on and some stud may allow a mocking minute of tension before the languid unknotting of the drawstring, and the peeling down of the tiny garment, freeing the cock and balls in one of the most mundane and heart-stopping moments there is.

An American guy, I thought, was doing this just now on the other side of the room; square and trim he stood breathing heavily and luxuriating under the water before turning his back and loosening his glittering briefs to reveal a firm hairless ass, milky white between the sun or sunbed-tanned zones of his back and thighs. I still had my really absurdly tiny black trunks on, and felt my cock protesting against their restraint, thickening up, and aching as it did so after the pounding it had lately been taking.

At first I used to feel embarrassed about getting a hard-on in the shower. But at the Corry much deliberate excitative soaping of cocks went on, and a number of members had their routine erections there each day. My own, though less regular, were, I think, hoped and looked out for.

~~~

THE EARLY TWENTIETH-CENTURY AMERICAN POET Amy Lowell wrote this rapturous ode to a female bather in which she stands, dazzling 'in a great burst of sunshine'.

'Woman, clad only in youth and in gallant perfection.'
'A Bather' by Amy Lowell[52]

After A Picture By Anders Zorn
Thick dappled by circles of sunshine and fluttering shade,
Your bright, naked body advances, blown over by leaves,

SENSATION: Swimming and Desire

Half-quenched in their various green, just a point of you showing,
A knee or a thigh, sudden glimpsed, then at once blotted into
The filmy and flickering forest, to start out again
Triumphant in smooth, supple roundness, edged sharp as white ivory,
Cool, perfect, with rose rarely tinting your lips and your breasts,
Swelling out from the green in the opulent curves of ripe fruit,
And hidden, like fruit, by the swift intermittence of leaves.
So, clinging to branches and moss, you advance on the ledges
Of rock which hang over the stream, with the wood-smells about you,
The pungence of strawberry plants, and of gum-oozing spruces,
While below runs the water, impatient, impatient — to take you,
To splash you, to run down your sides, to sing you of deepness,
Of pools brown and golden, with brown-and-gold flags on their borders,
Of blue, lingering skies floating solemnly over your beauty,
Of undulant waters a-sway in the effort to hold you,
To keep you submerged and quiescent while over you glories
The Summer.
Oread, Dryad, or Naiad, or just
Woman, clad only in youth and in gallant perfection,
Standing up in a great burst of sunshine, you dazzle my eyes
Like a snow-star, a moon, your effulgence burns up in a halo,
For you are the chalice which holds all the races of men.

You slip into the pool and the water folds over your shoulder,

And over the tree-tops the clouds slowly follow your swimming,
And the scent of the woods is sweet on this hot Summer morning.

CHAPTER III

Old Times

EROTIC ENCOUNTERS ON THE BEACH or in the pool have been written about since ancient times. In *The Arabian Nights*, the conceit is that the king is planning to put the storyteller, Scheherazade, to death in the morning. But her cliffhanger endings are so compelling that, each time, he decides to postpone her execution until he hears the next episode. So the narrator of the original, anonymous text is imagined to be female – but this is simply a device for stringing stories together.

This translation by Richard Francis Burton first appeared in 1885. Burton, an Anglo-Irish army officer, linguist and explorer with a strong interest in sex, has been criticised for over-emphasising the erotic content of the source material, which dates from the Islamic Golden Age of the eighth to thirteenth centuries. Released in a subscriber-only edition to skirt around the UK's obscenity laws, it was a highly prized addition to the 'Naughty' section of private libraries in the late nineteenth century. It's probably the case that most readily available translations veer in the other direction – censoring rather than enhancing the original.

'She threw herself into the basin, and swam and dived.'

'The Book of the Thousand Nights and a Night', *A Plain and Literal Translation of the Arabian Nights Entertainments* by Richard Francis Burton[53]

The Ninth Night

Once upon a time there was a Porter in Baghdad. It came to pass on a certain day, as he stood about the street leaning idly upon his crate, behold, there stood before him an honourable woman in a mantilla of Mosul silk, broidered with gold and bordered with brocade; She raised her face-veil and, showing two black eyes fringed with jetty lashes, whose glances were soft and languishing and whose perfect beauty was ever blandishing, she accosted the Porter and said in the suavest tones and choicest language.

'Take up thy crate and follow me.' The Porter was so dazzled he could hardly believe that he heard her aright, but he shouldered his basket in hot haste saying in himself,

'O day of good luck! O day of Allah's grace!' and walked after her till she stopped at the door of a house. There she rapped, and presently came out to her an old man, a Nazarene, to whom she gave a gold piece, receiving from him in return what she required of strained wine clear as olive oil; and she set it safely in the hamper, saying,

'Lift and follow.'

Quoth the Porter, 'This, by Allah, is indeed an auspicious day, a day propitious for the granting of all a man wisheth.' He again hoisted up the crate and followed her; till she stopped at a fruiterer's shop and bought from him Shámi apples and Osmáni quinces and Omani peaches, and cucumbers of Nile growth, and Egyptian limes and Sultáni oranges and citrons; besides Aleppine jasmine, scented myrtle berries,

Damascene nenuphars, flower of privet and camomile, blood-red anemones, violets, and pomegranate-bloom, eglantine and narcissus, and set the whole in the Porter's crate, saying, 'Up with it.'

The Porter follows her into a mansion where he ends up partying with the lady and her two sisters.

Then the lady took the cup, and drank it off to her sisters' health, and they ceased-not drinking (the Porter being in the midst of them), and dancing and laughing and reciting verses and singing ballads and ritornellos. All this time the Porter was carrying on with them, kissing, toying, biting, handling, groping, fingering; whilst one thrust a dainty morsel in his mouth, and another slapped him; and this cuffed his cheeks, and that threw sweet flowers at him; and he was in the very paradise of pleasure, as though he were sitting in the seventh sphere among the Houris of Heaven.

They ceased-not doing after this fashion until the wine played tricks in their heads and worsted their wits; and, when the drink got the better of them, the portress stood up and doffed her clothes till she was mother-naked. However, she let down her hair about her body by way of shift, and throwing herself into the basin disported herself and dived like a duck and swam up and down, and took water in her mouth, and spurted it all over the Porter, and washed her limbs, and between her breasts, and inside her thighs and all around her navel.

Then she came up out of the cistern and throwing herself on the Porter's lap said,

'O my lord, O my love, what callest thou this article?' pointing to her slit, her solution of continuity.

'I call that thy cleft,' quoth the Porter, and she rejoined,

'Wah! wah! art thou not ashamed to use such a word?' and she caught him by the collar and soundly cuffed him.

Said he again, 'Thy womb, thy vulva;' and she struck him a second slap crying,

'O fie, O fie, this is another ugly word; is there no shame in thee?'

Quoth he, 'Thy coynte;' and she cried,

'O thou! art wholly destitute of modesty?' and thumped him and bashed him.

Then cried the Porter, 'Thy clitoris,' whereat the eldest lady came down upon him with a yet sorer beating, and said,

'No;' and he said,

''Tis so,' and the Porter went on calling the same commodity by sundry other names, but whatever he said they beat him more and more till his neck ached and swelled with the blows he had gotten; and on this wise they made him a butt and a laughing-stock.

Then the cateress donned her clothes and they fell again to carousing, but the Porter kept moaning, 'Oh! and Oh!' for his neck and shoulders, and the cup passed merrily round and round again for a full hour. After that time the eldest and handsomest lady stood up and stripped off her garments. Then she threw herself into the basin, and swam and dived, sported and washed; and the Porter looked at her naked figure as though she had been a slice of the moon and at her face with the sheen of Luna when at full, or like the dawn when it brighteneth, and he noted her noble stature and shape, and those glorious forms that quivered as she went; for she was naked as the Lord made her. Then he cried,

'Alack! Alack!' and began to address her, versifying in these couplets:—

'If I liken thy shape to the bough when green

My likeness errs and I sore mistake it;
For the bough is fairest when clad the most
And thou art fairest when mother-naked.'

~~~

THE WATERSIDE FLIRTATION HERE DESCRIBED is even older; it is one in which Plutarch tells an illuminating anecdote about Cleopatra, the last active ruler of the Ptolemaic Kingdom of Egypt from 51 to 30 BCE.

'He ordered the fisherman to dive under the water.'

Marcus Antonius, Plutarch's Lives (translated from Greek by Aubrey Stewart and George Long)[54]

Though Cleopatra received many letters of summons both from Antonius and his friends, she so despised and mocked the man, that she sailed up the Cydnus in a vessel with a gilded stern, with purple sails spread, and rowers working with silver oars to the sound of the flute in harmony with pipes and lutes. Cleopatra reclined under an awning spangled with gold, dressed as Venus is painted, and youths representing the Cupids in pictures stood on each side fanning her. In like manner the handsomest of her female slaves in the dress of Nereids and Graces, were stationed some at the rudders and others at the ropes. And odours of wondrous kind from much incense filled the banks. Some of the people accompanied her immediately from the entrance of the river on both sides, and others went down from the city to see the sight . . .

Now her beauty, as they say, was not in itself altogether incomparable nor such as to strike those who saw her; but familiarity with her had an irresistible charm, and her form, combined with her persuasive speech and with the peculiar character which in a manner was diffused about her behaviour, produced a certain piquancy. There was a sweetness also in the sound of her voice when she spoke; and as she could easily turn her tongue, like a many-stringed instrument, to any language that she pleased, she had very seldom need of an interpreter for her communication with barbarians, but she answered most by herself.

Cleopatra, by distributing flattery not, as Plato says in four ways, but in many ways, and by always adding some new pleasure and charm to whatever was either serious or mirthful, completely ruled Antonius, never leaving him by night nor by day. For she played at dice with him, and drank with him, and hunted with him, and was a spectator when he was exercising in arms, and by night when he was standing at the doors and windows of the common people and jesting with those within, she accompanied him in his rambles and freaks, in the dress of a female slave; for Antonius also used to dress himself in this style . . .

On one occasion when he was fishing and was vexed at his bad sport, Cleopatra also being present, he ordered the fisherman to dive under the water and secretly to fasten to the hook some fishes that had been already caught; and he pulled up two or three times, but not without being detected by the Egyptian.

Pretending to admire, she spoke to her friends and invited them to come as spectators on the following day. A number of them got into the fishing boats, and when Antonius had let down his line, she ordered one of her own men to anticipate him by diving to the hook and to fasten to it a Pontic salted fish. Antonius thinking that he had caught something pulled up, on which there was, as was natural, great laughter, whereat Cleopatra said, 'Give up the fishing-rod, Imperator, to us the kings of Pharos and Canopus; your sport is cities and kings and continents.'

CHAPTER IV

The Male Gaze

WHEN IT COMES TO WOMEN swimming, what's called 'the male gaze' (a concept first articulated by British feminist film theorist Laura Mulvey in 1975) has long been hard at work, especially at the water's edge. In bygone days, gents would roam beach resorts, telescopes in hand, to catch a glimpse of uncovered flesh. Charles Sprawson in his 1992 celebration of the 'swimmer as hero', *Haunts of the Black Masseur*, quotes novelist John Cowper Powys, himself a voyeur, noting: 'Elderly gentlemen, betrayed by their curiously high-coloured faces, as if they lived on the heart's blood of women, as they hunted and stared and eternally stared and hunted.'

The perspective from which we see female characters in writing about swimming – at the beach, in the pool, on the river's edge – is often the same wherever they appear. A friend who reads for a publishing house says almost all of the manuscripts she receives by male writers offer an assessment, entirely unasked-for, of the attractiveness of every female character – from the murder victim to the sentencing judge, from the midwife to the barista. This seemingly instinctive trope lurks even in the best of writing.

This charming Chekhov story 'Gooseberries' is the tale behind the title of George Saunders's book, *A Swim in a Pond in the Rain*, about how learning and teaching Russian short stories has informed his life.

'Gooseberries' opens with two men on a hunting trip. They visit a farmer friend and go for a swim. One of the trio has a tale to tell – about going on a visit to the brother he loved dearly as a child, only to discover that he has become a smug landowner with dubious politics.

It is a masterpiece which Saunders justly raves about. But for a feminist reader, the fact that Saunders doesn't even notice the petty sexism of this exchange with the maid Pelagueya is frustrating. She brings the men soap and towels when they go swimming, and her prettiness is a pivotal moment. She is so attractive that, on meeting her, both of the visitors stop and exchange glances. (That's right, they exchange glances not with Pelagueya but with each other.)

'In the middle of the pool he lay on his back to let the rain fall on his face.'
'Gooseberries' by Anton Chekhov[55]

The house was large and two-storied. Aliokhin lived downstairs in two vaulted rooms with little windows designed for the farmhands; the farmhouse was plain, and the place smelled of rye bread and vodka, and leather. He rarely used the reception-rooms, only when guests arrived. Ivan Ivanich and Bourkin were received by a chambermaid; such a pretty young woman that both of them stopped and exchanged glances.

'You cannot imagine how glad I am to see you, gentlemen,' said Aliokhin, coming after them into the hall. 'I never expected you. Pelagueya,' he said to the maid, 'give my friends a change of clothes. And I will change, too. But I must have a bath. I haven't had one since the spring. Wouldn't you like to come to the bathing shed? And meanwhile our things will be got ready.'

Pretty Pelagueya, dainty and sweet, brought towels and soap, and Aliokhin led his guests to the bathing-shed. 'Yes,' he said, 'it is a long time since I had a bath. My bathing-shed is all right, as you see. My father and I put it up, but somehow I have no time to bathe.'

He sat down on the step and lathered his long hair and neck, and the water round him became brown.

'Yes. I see,' said Ivan Ivanich heavily, looking at his head. 'It is a long time since I bathed,' said Aliokhin shyly, as he soaped himself again, and the water round him became dark blue, like ink. Ivan Ivanich came out of the shed, plunged into the water with a splash, and swam about in the rain, flapping his arms, and sending waves back, and on the waves tossed white lilies; he swam out to the middle of the pool and dived, and in a minute came up again in another place and kept on swimming and diving, trying to reach the bottom.

'Ah! how delicious!' he shouted in his glee. 'How delicious!' He swam to the mill, spoke to the peasants, and came back, and in the middle of the pool he lay on his back to let the rain fall on his face. Bourkin and Aliokin were already dressed and ready to go, but he kept on swimming and diving.

'Delicious,' he said. 'Too delicious!'

'You've had enough,' shouted Bourkin.

WE DON'T FIND OUT WHAT Pelagueya thought here. But the perspective of a woman is often assumed to be quite narcissistic – to the extent that she experiences desire, that desire is focused on attracting the powerful male gaze to her.

In another story by Anton Chekhov, the novella, *The Duel*, bathing is a daily habit in the heat of summer in a Black Sea village where the central character Ivan Andreitch Laevsky has moved to live with his married lover. The opening scene seems to me very like what we call these days, in Scotland, a bob and a blether. A group of men – I enjoy imagining them as like our local Edinburgh Blueballs – discuss matters of love in the water.

'The man sitting at the helm looked at her, and she liked being looked at . . .'
The Duel by Anton Chekhov[56]

It was eight o'clock in the morning – the time when the officers, the local officials, and the visitors usually took their morning dip in the sea after the hot, stifling night, and then went into the pavilion to drink tea or coffee. Ivan Andreitch Laevsky, a thin, fair young man of twenty-eight, wearing the cap of a clerk in the Ministry of Finance and with slippers on his feet, coming down to bathe, found a number of acquaintances on the beach, and among them his friend Samoylenko, the army doctor.

'Answer one question for me, Alexandr Daviditch,' Laevsky began, when both he and Samoylenko were in the water up to their shoulders. 'Suppose you had loved a woman and had been living with her for two or three years, and then left off caring for her, as one does, and began to feel that you had nothing in common with her. How would you behave in that case?'

'It's very simple. "You go where you please, madam" – and that would be the end of it.'

'It's easy to say that! But if she has nowhere to go? A woman with no friends or relations, without a farthing, who can't work . . .'

'Well? Five hundred roubles down or an allowance of twenty-five roubles a month – and nothing more. It's very simple.'

'Even supposing you have five hundred roubles and can pay twenty-five roubles a month, the woman I am speaking of is an educated woman and proud. Could you really bring yourself to offer her money? And how would you do it?'

Samoylenko was going to answer, but at that moment a big wave covered them both, then broke on the beach and rolled back noisily over the shingle. The friends got out and began dressing

'Of course, it is difficult to live with a woman if you don't love her,' said Samoylenko, shaking the sand out of his boots. 'But one must look at the thing humanely, Vanya. If it were my case, I should never show a sign that I did not love her, and I should go on living with her till I died.'

He was at once ashamed of his own words; he pulled himself up and said:

'But for aught I care, there might be no females at all. Let them all go to the devil!'

The friends dressed and went into the pavilion. There Samoylenko was quite at home, and even had a special cup and saucer. Every morning they brought him on a tray a cup of coffee, a tall cut glass of iced water, and a tiny glass of brandy. He would first drink the brandy, then the hot coffee, then the iced water, and this must have been very nice, for after drinking it his eyes looked moist with pleasure, he would stroke his whiskers with both hands, and say, looking at the sea:

'A wonderfully magnificent view!'

Laevsky has fallen so out of love with Nadyezhda Fyodorovna that all he can think of is how to escape. Meanwhile, Nadyezhda has her own admirers and has had a brief, regretted, dalliance with the local police captain. She regards herself as the most beautiful woman in the town. Though the men dip in the open sea, the women are generally confined to a bath house. At one point, while there, Nadyezhda and her companions see a fourteen-year-old boy showing off and then becoming exhausted in the nearby waters.

Nadyezhda Fyodorovna put on her straw hat and dashed out into the open sea. She swam some thirty feet and then turned on her back. She could see the sea to the horizon, the steamers, the people on the sea-front, the town; and all this, together with the sultry heat and the soft, transparent waves, excited her and whispered that she must live, live . . . A sailing-boat darted by her rapidly and vigorously, cleaving the waves and the air; the man sitting at the helm looked at her, and she liked being looked at . . .

~~~

THE VOYEURISTIC GOGGLES ARE FIRMLY in place, too, in F. Scott Fitzgerald's 1929 short story 'The Swimmers'. Married man Henry Marston watches a young American woman enter the water on a beach, and is so enchanted that when she gets into trouble, he tries to rescue her in spite of not being able to swim. It's this unfortunate escapade that takes him on a journey of learning how to swim that will transform his life.

'The burden of his wretched marriage fell away with the buoyant tumble of his body among the swells.'
'The Swimmers' by F. Scott Fitzgerald[57]

The girl – she was perhaps eighteen – was obviously acting like nothing but herself – she was what his father would have called a thoroughbred. A deep, thoughtful face that was pretty only because of the irrepressible determination of the perfect features to be recognized, a face that could have done without them and not yielded up its poise and distinction.

In her grace, at once exquisite and hardy, she was that perfect type of American girl that makes one wonder if the male is not being sacrificed to it, much as, in the last century, the lower strata in England were sacrificed to produce the governing class.

The two young men, coming out of the water as she went in, had large shoulders and empty faces. She had a smile for them that was no more than they deserved – that must do until she chose one to be the father of her children and gave herself up to destiny. Until then – Henry Marston was glad about her as her arms, like flying fish, clipped the water in a crawl, as her body spread in a swan dive or doubled in a jackknife from the springboard and her head appeared from the depth, jauntily flipping the damp hair away.

The two young men passed near.

"They push water," Choupette said, "then they go elsewhere and push other water. They pass months in France and they couldn't tell you the name of the President. They are parasites such as Europe has not known in a hundred years."

But Henry had stood up abruptly, and now all the people on the beach were suddenly standing up. Something had happened out there in the fifty yards between the deserted raft and the shore. The bright head showed upon the surface; it did not flip water now, but called: "Au secours! Help!" in a feeble and frightened voice.

"Henry!" Choupette cried. "Stop! Henry!"

The beach was almost deserted at noon, but Henry and several others were sprinting toward the sea; the two young Americans heard, turned and sprinted after them. There was a frantic little time with half a dozen bobbing heads in the water. Choupette, still clinging to her parasol, but managing to wring her hands at the same time, ran up and down the beach crying: "Henry! Henry!"

Now there were more helping hands, and then two swelling groups around prostrate figures on the shore. The young fellow who pulled in the girl brought her around in a minute or so, but they had more trouble getting the water out of Henry, who had never learned to swim.

The girl, saved, begins, the next day to teach Henry to swim, and the water becomes his place of retreat, solace and rejuvenation.

When difficulties became insurmountable, inevitable, Henry sought surcease in exercise. For three years, swimming had been a sort of refuge, and he turned to it as one man to music or another to drink. There was a point when he would resolutely stop thinking and go to the Virginia coast for a week to wash his mind in the water. Far out past the breakers he could survey the green-and-brown line of the Old Dominion with the pleasant impersonality of a porpoise. The burden of his wretched marriage fell away with the buoyant tumble of his body among the swells, and he would begin to move in a child's dream of space. Sometimes remembered playmates of his youth swam with him; sometimes, with his two sons beside him, he seemed to be setting off along the bright pathway to the moon. Americans, he liked to say, should be born with fins, and perhaps they were – perhaps money was a form of fin. In England property begot a strong place sense, but Americans, restless and with shallow roots, needed fins and wings.

CHAPTER V

Sexy Beasts

YOU DON'T HAVE TO BE human to be sexy. The mythological creatures and spirits inhabiting waters – sirens, mermaids, sprites – would often be characterised as having an allure, sometimes deadly, and not infrequently find themselves portrayed through a male gaze.

Waters, and their spirits, are places of enticement. The great Russian poet Alexander Pushkin told of a hermit monk lured into the water by a water nymph. Such nymphs, or water deities, have cast a spell over mythology for millennia. Pushkin was inspired by the Rusalka of Slavic folklore, originally bringers of fertility, although in the nineteenth century these water dwellers were recast as malicious and dangerous pranksters.

'Into the water like a shooting star.'
'The Water-Nymph' by Alexander Pushkin[58]

> In lakeside leafy groves, a friar
> Escaped all worries; there he passed
> His summer days in constant prayer,
> Deep studies and eternal fast.

SENSATION: Swimming and Desire

Already with a humble shovel
The elder dug himself a grave –
As, calling saints to bless his hovel,
Death – nothing other – did he crave.

So once, upon a falling night, he
Was bowing by his wilted shack
With meekest prayer to the Almighty.
The grove was turning slowly black;
Above the lake a mist was lifting;
Through milky clouds across the sky
The ruddy moon was softly drifting,
When water drew the friar's eye . . .

He's looking puzzled, full of trouble,
A fear he cannot quite explain,
He sees the waves begin to bubble
And suddenly grow calm again.
Then – white as first snow in the highlands,
Light-footed as nocturnal shade,
There comes ashore, and sits in silence
Upon the bank, a naked maid.

She eyes the monk and brushes gently
Her hair, and water off her arms.
He shakes with fear and looks intently
At her, and at her lovely charms.
With eager hand she waves and beckons,
Nods quickly, smiles as from afar

And flies, within two flashing seconds,
Into the water like a shooting star.

The glum old man slept not an instant;
All day, not even once he prayed:
Before his eyes still hung and glistened
The wondrous, the relentless shade . . .
The grove puts on its gown of nightfall;
The moon walks on the cloudy floor;
And there's the maiden – pale, delightful,
Reclining on the spellbound shore.

She looks at him, her hair she brushes,
Blows airy kisses, gestures wild,
Plays with the waves – caresses, splashes –
Now laughs, now whimpers like a child,
Moans tenderly, calls louder, louder . . .
'Come, monk, come, monk! To me, to me!'
Then – disappears in limpid water,
And all is silent instantly . . .

On the third day the zealous hermit
Was sitting by the shore, in love,
Awaiting the delightful mermaid,
As shade was covering the grove . . .
Dark ceded to the sun's emergence;
Our monk had wholly disappeared –
Before a crowd of local urchins,
Fishing, found his grey foam beard.

Pushkin's wood nymph is, for all its deep roots in Slavic mythology, also a creature of a time, portrayed by a man at a nineteenth-century moment when it seemed the arts were teeming with half-naked nymphs, fairies and other figures often ogled in a romanticised, yet dubious way. Some of these works now come with a slight cringe – for instance, pre-Raphaelite John William Waterhouse's 'Hylas and the Nymphs', in which seven topless and adolescent female forms seduce the tragic Argonaut. But was it a publicity stunt or genuine outrage that in 2018 led Manchester Art Gallery to remove the image from its walls for seven days?

Not all female figures are there to entice, however. Some are finding their own rapture. It would be neglectful not to mention a particular strand of marine erotica featuring tentacled monsters and the female divers.

Most famous is a woodcut from the nineteenth century by the great Japanese artist Hokusai. 'The Dream of the Fisherman's Wife' or 'The Shelldiver and Two Octopi' shows a woman apparently being pleasured by two octopi. It has been interpreted and misinterpreted in various ways. As the art historian Matthi Forrer points out in his biography, the sense of humour of working-class Japanese culture from two centuries ago is pretty much a closed book to us, but we know Hokusai was regarded as a wit. Seeing the similarity between the face of the octopus and the male figure in other erotic wood carvings, it seems that Hokusai may be suggesting that, as far as the fisherman's wife goes, the best lover imaginable might be an octopus.

CHAPTER VI

Free From the Gaze

WHAT'S BEEN INTERESTING IN RECENT years is to see how wild swimming culture has often offered a refuge from this judgemental or even predatory male gaze (even if just because, in the winter months, the wind and wild weather keep all but those focused on the water away).

Yes, there are still beaches, where men, in the words of The Stranglers, while away their hours looking at the 'Peaches', and women do their own watching of the beefcakes, or whoever, in terms of gender or form, most catches the eye. And there are, too, men who belong to swimming groups who speak of body positivity and the water's role in banishing self-consciousness.

But what I've found is that a lot of swimmers resolutely reject the idea of the 'beach body'. In my years spent interviewing wild swimmers, I've come to realise that women in particular have built together a place and a community where how you look really doesn't matter too much.

One swimmer, Angela Weir, described how she discovered swimming around the same time as her (now ex) husband told her, pointing at her body, that he didn't want to be with 'this' anymore.

'I find,' she said, 'that there is no judgement, no body shaming, and I have never felt conscious of my size down at Wardie Bay. It has done so much for my body confidence and my general confidence and, on those down days, you just swim a wee bit further out and have a wee cry. The water soothes and holds me, and I go home feeling ready for anything.'

Some swimmers, including myself, embrace throwing aside modesty and going for the occasional skinny dip. For so many of us, a naked swim in the sea is a genuinely liberating way to strip off those awkward thermal layers of self-consciousness. One of the recent authors who describes that particular freedom best is Ruth Fitzmaurice.

'Cold water gives us new skin.'
I Found My Tribe by Ruth Fitzmaurice[59]

Sea swimming does wonders for your inhibitions. For the first few weeks I cowered self-consciously on the cove steps. My baby-battered body felt exposed. These days we shed clothes like discarded sweet wrappers. The packaging is incidental. We climb out of the water like mermaid goddesses. Cold water gives us new skin.

OF COURSE TO GO NAKED, or to strip down to a sturdy, 'bits'-covering swimsuit is not what all women want or need. That's not necessarily the point. It was not, for instance, what a group of Somali women learning to open water swim – who are featured in my co-authored book *The Ripple Effect* – were looking for. Rather, that was to find a body of water 'not too public or overlooked'. Plus a good set of donated wetsuits.

Wetsuit or birthday suit, the best of wild swimming culture for women prioritises activity and enjoyment of one's body over what anyone wears, or doesn't. The emphasis on body positivity is ubiquitous – and perhaps one of the most empowering advocates for this is the *Outdoor Swimmer* editor, Ella Foote, who refuses to allow her sporting ability to be judged in terms of her weight.

'Suddenly I am worthy of his attention, respect. I put my head down and keep swimming.'

'An open letter to every plus-size swimmer who's afraid of being mocked at the pool' by Ella Foote[60]

I am stood in a swimsuit, swim cap and goggles waiting for the rest of the group I am with to get their wetsuits on so we can tackle a one kilometre sea swim. They have just run six kilometres of the brutal Exmoor coastal path; I hitched a lift with the event organisers. I am on a press trip, but it is being hosted by an adventure company, so the others are not the usual media types. I try to make small talk with the guy next to me. I ask him if we had met before as he seems familiar. He looks me up and down before saying he very much doubts it.

'Are you going in like that?' another chap exclaims. 'You're going to be really cold.'

I smile and politely reassure him that I will be okay, while he exchanges looks with the other guy. I have been in this position many times, at the start of many swimming events. Seasoned, regular outdoor swimmers know, you simply cannot judge a swimmer by their body.

We stand side by side. The group have bonded on their shared experience on the run, understanding each other better, knowing who is capable of what. I knew I wouldn't have been able to keep up on the run, my body and I know each other well. Now at the water's edge, the one kilometre sea swim ahead isn't a challenge, it is a joy. The anticipation is more based on excitement. As soon as I am into the blue, I am at ease, I am held, I swim. It isn't fast, with lots of effort. Just strong and consistent, the way I have taught my body. The lead safety guy asks me to hang back for the rest of the group to catch up. The man I had tried to chat to swims up behind, wearing fins.

'I don't think we have properly met,' he offers. 'Are you some sort of cold water swimmer or something?'

Suddenly I am worthy of his attention, respect. I put my head down and keep swimming.

It isn't the first time I have surprised others once in the water. I work hard at the start of any big swim not to let the people around me get into my head. There is a great feeling swimming past someone who gave unsolicited advice or concern before starting. But why does it have to happen in the first place?

The media loves a statistic about obesity and can fuel stigma towards people who are overweight. Anyone who does any kind of activity regularly knows that just because someone may look 'fit' it doesn't mean that they are. While I applaud and admire a person who can love their body at any size, I can't find peace with mine. So I seek activity to address the problem, build strength and health the best I can – don't shame me before I have begun.

Fashion Blogger Chloe Elliott can relate, also falling victim to assumptions when she took up ballet. 'It was immediately assumed by the instructor that I was less able,' she says. 'I was told I could alter movements to make them "easier" for me. It was frustrating that it was automatically assumed I was less capable because of my size, when there were people half my size, less flexible than me and they were treated normally.'

This year I signed up to a nine kilometre river swim, my first proper event swim in three years. I have longer distances on my swim CV, but I am the biggest I have ever been and so the shame surrounding my body is worse than ever. It doesn't really matter if I finish or not, but I did find myself saying to a friend that it is different when a fat person fails at sport. Because if I get fished out the water half-way, it is because of my weight. If a 'fit' looking person gets fished out, it's misadventure, bad luck, lack of training.

As a swimming journalist, I was recently interviewing ocean swim-mer Beth French. Beth set out to swim the Oceans Seven, a challenge consisting of the seven most dangerous sea-channels in the world; a film has been made about her story. I asked her experience of failure and success. 'My goal was to swim seven oceans in a year, that was the desti-nation,' she says. 'But the adventure is what we learn along the way and that is why we do it. We don't do these swims, challenges and projects for the end result, we do it for what we learn about ourselves during the process.' Her words stuck with me. Never has any big swim for me been about placing my feet back onto dry land at the end.

Both Ella and the remarkable Beth French (who wrote her bucket list of big swims as a wheelchair user and while suffering from ME) are powerful role models who remind us how there is no perfect swim body, and that the athletic, or even the simply capable body, comes in many forms.

The great thing, too, is that there is no need as a swimmer to think you, and your body, are past it. Some of the most challenging swims have been conquered relatively late in life. Perhaps most famous of these is Diana Nyad's crawl through shark- and jellyfish-infested waters from Cuba to Florida, achieved on her fifth attempt at sixty-four years old.

The story of her long-running battle, begun with a first attempt at the age of twenty-four, has been told both in an inspiring biopic starring Annette Bening, and in Nyad's memoir, *Finding A Way*. On reaching Key West, face puffed, lips chapped and struggling to stand, Nyad famously said, 'I have three messages. One is, we should never, ever give up. Two is, you're never too old to chase your dream. Three is, it looks like a solitary sport, but it is a team.'

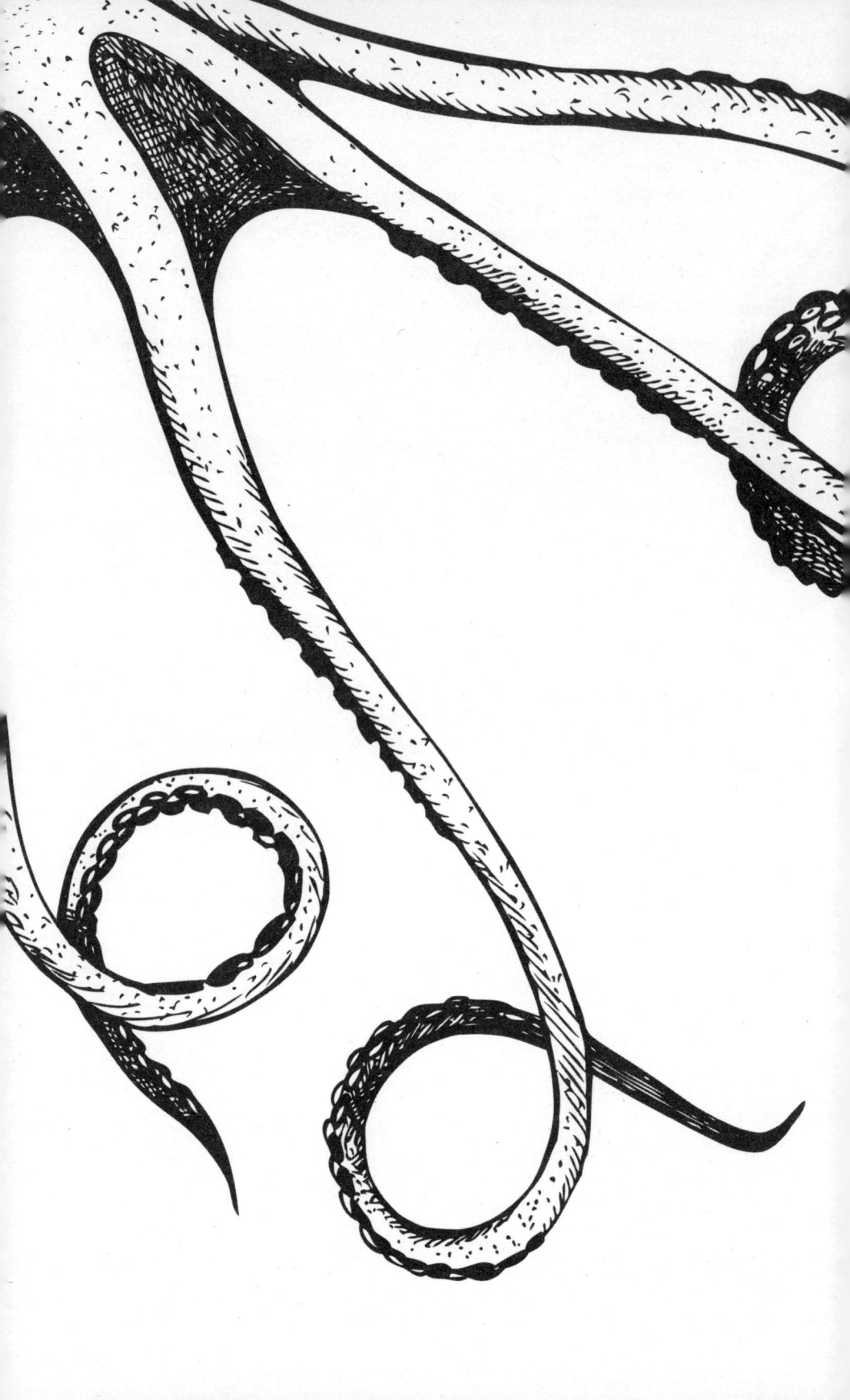

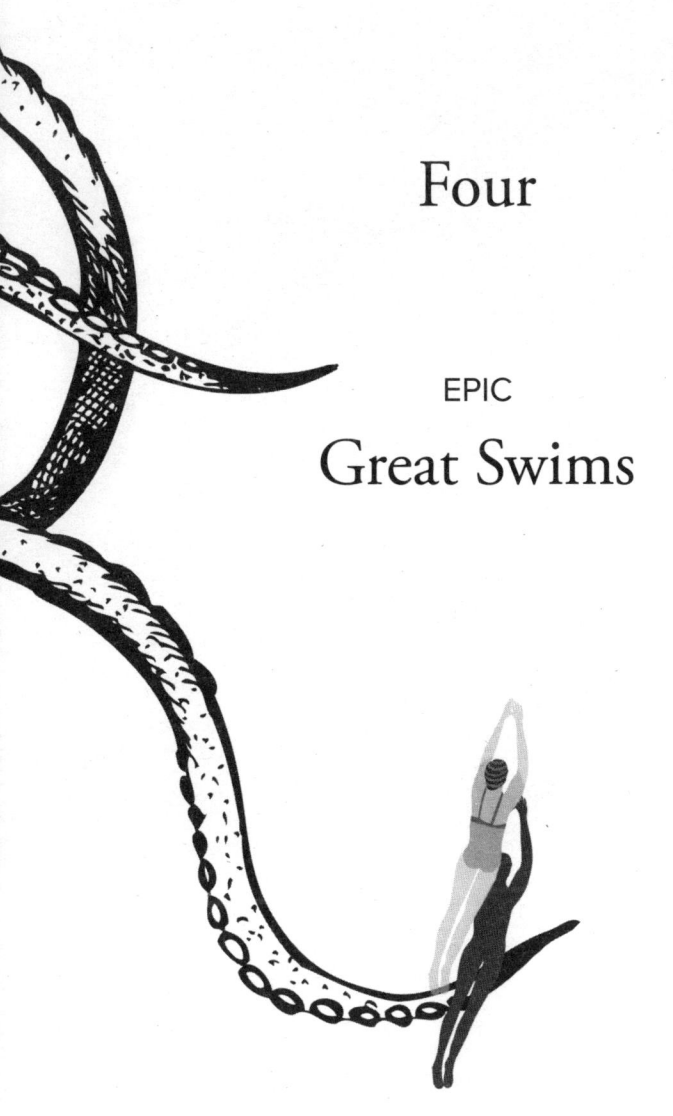

Four

EPIC

Great Swims

'NOTHING GREAT IS EASY,' IS THE LINE ENGRAVED on English Channel swimmer Captain Matthew Webb's memorial.

Myself, I'm not a long-distance swimmer; I'm what they call a dipper. But whenever I have been far from the shore on, for instance, a memorable longer swim, from the Hebridean isle of Lewis to the captivating Pabbay island, I think of the heroes. I think of those who have set forth on the sea with nothing more than their arms, legs and the twisting propellor of their body. I marvel at what it must take to tough it out over miles, in extreme cold, rough seas or jellyfish-infested waters. I think of the true legends – Lynne Cox, Diana Nyad, Mercedes Gleitze, Lewis Pugh, Captain Webb, Gertrude Ederle, Pablo Fernandez. I think of those I have dipped with who have swum far and long – Cath Pendleton, Alice Goodridge.

History is littered with iconic swims and tales of the heroes who have made them. Their endurance creates a kind of slipstream. You don't have to swim the Channel to feel a touch of their inspiration, of their fortitude and perseverance. You can carry their words inside your head on a swim across the bay, or you can simply let them sit there shoreside as you imagine following in their strokes one day.

CHAPTER I

Cold Waters, Cold Wars

I CONFESS, AS AN ENVIRONMENTAL journalist, I reserve particular admiration for Lewis Pugh, who uses his powers of swimming to high-light the climate crisis. He has made swimming into a form of activism, using it to attract attention to the urgent problems of climate change and our human impact on natural waters.

Ahead of a swim he did in 2020 in Antarctica, I spoke to Pugh, the UN Patron of the Oceans, about his 'Speedo diplomacy', which has taken him to swim in Arctic waters, the 315-mile length of the Hudson River and across glacial Lake Pumori on Mount Everest, which was the 'highest' ever endurance swim.

Pugh's 2020 swim was done as part of a bid to negotiate the creation of a network of marine-protected areas around Antarctica, and was one in which, Pugh said, 'You know you are on the edge of life and death.'

'I'm fifty now,' he said, 'and the science is very clear. The older you get, the less tolerant you get to cold water. But I'm so determined to get Antarctica protected. My determination is stronger than the indifference of any nation.'

Pugh had swum in such extremes before. He recalled, for instance, a 350-metre swim across a stretch of the Ross Sea where the water temperature was just below zero but the air much colder. He recalled: 'You take your arm from –1.7°C and push it into –37°C – so you just want to pull it out to warm it back up.

Pugh has written several books, including the intriguingly titled *21 Yaks and a Speedo – How to Achieve Your Impossible*, and also publishes a compelling online journal (at lewispugh.com). In this powerful blog, from 3 September 2021, he writes about a lengthy swim he made in the icy waters off Greenland, across the Ilulissat Icefjord, which is fed by the world's fastest-moving glacier.

'I'm freezing here, to remind world leaders that if we push our planet too far, all our lives are at risk.'
'A World of Difference' by Lewis Pugh[61]

They say three is a magic number. When it comes to temperature, I know this to be true. For a cold-water swimmer, a 3°C change makes a world of difference. The same is true for our planet.

Before I started on this Greenland swim I was hoping for an average water temperature of 3°C. But when we arrived at Ilulissat the water temperature was 0°C. We had to change my swim plan.

This is different from anything I've done before. Instead of a one-kilometre sprint, it's 7.8 kilometres over multiple days. The effects of cold are cumulative, so we decided to split each day's distance into two shorter swims, rather than one longer one, to give me time to re-warm my body in between.

Pugh goes on to describe his elaborate preparations, the precautions taken and the very real threat of hypothermia, before returning to a description of the swim . . .

All of these preparations involve things we can control. But Mother Nature makes her own plans. Each day in Ilulissat has brought new challenges. A strong mind is as important as peak physical condition, but it can't be so strong as to override your survival instinct – the pain is telling you that you're in danger. It's a fine line.

As we have crossed halfway, I'm certainly feeling the effects of the cold. My body is sore. And at night I keep asking myself how much longer I can keep this up. But somehow I'll keep going; I've got a very good reason to.

When it comes to our heating planet, we don't have a three-degree margin. Scientists tell us that a 2°C increase above pre-industrial temperatures will push us past a point of no return. The latest IPCC report suggests that we have already exceeded 1.5°C.

Our Earth evolved as a complex living system in delicate balance. In the same way that I need to make adjustments to my body to deal with the extreme cold, we need to make serious changes to stop our planet from heating up any further.

I'm freezing here, to remind world leaders that if we push our planet too far, all our lives are at risk.

There is a world of difference in just 2°C. Let's not put this number to the ultimate test.

<hr/>

LONG-DISTANCE SWIMMER LYNNE COX HAS been credited for easing the Cold War tensions between Ronald Reagan and Mikhail Gorbachev when she symbolically linked them by becoming the first person to swim between the USA and the Soviet Union. On 7 August 1987, she braved the frigid waters of the Bering Strait to swim 2.3 miles from the island of Little Diomede in Alaska to Big Diomede, which was then part of the Soviet Union. At the time, the reality of the Cold War meant the Inuit were forbidden to travel between the islands.

At the signing of the INF Missile Treaty at the White House later that year, Gorbachev made a toast. He and President Reagan lifted their glasses and Gorbachev said: 'Last summer it took one brave American by the name of Lynne Cox just two hours to swim from one of our countries to the other. We saw on television how sincere and friendly the meeting was between our people and the Americans when she stepped onto the Soviet shore. She proved by her courage how close to each other our peoples live.'

'The Soviet people are waiting for you.'
Swimming to Antarctica by Lynne Cox[62]

Turning to breathe, I saw the crew of the Soviet launch pointing to a snowbank a half mile south of us. Vladimir McMillian, the man with the curly brown hair, shouted excitedly to me,

'The Soviet people are waiting for you over there. They could not manage to climb down these cliffs. But they would like to meet and see you at the finish.'

'Lynne, you can stop now,' Dr Keatinge shouted. His voice was heavy with concern. He was afraid that my temperature would drop more. He hadn't been able to get a reading.

'You know, if you stop now, you will have succeeded,' Dr Keatinge said.

'How far is the snowbank?' I asked.

Vladimir asked a crewman, then told me, 'Half a mile.'

'Bill, it's okay if I stop now?' I asked Dr Keatinge, trying to decide what to do.

'Yes. Yes. You can finish right there,' he said, pointing to a rock.

We were fifty yards from our goal.

'She's heading into shore,' I heard Dr Keatinge say, his voice filled with relief.

But when I turned to breathe, I saw the bright snow on the beach and I saw the little black dots that must have been the Soviet people standing there. I asked myself, *Will you be satisfied if you stop now? Everything you have done has been about extending yourself, about going beyond borders. You've had to go beyond your physical and psychological borders. Everything everyone has done for you and for themselves to this point has been about extending themselves, too, beyond their own borders, about believing when there was little to believe in.*

But now you can stop. You're only ten yards from shore. You can stop now and know that you have succeeded.

God, I want to. I've got to think about how cold I'm going to be when I climb out of the water. I took a few more strokes forward. You've got to decide now, I told myself. In a moment the crew will be preparing to land.

'You can finish on that rock,' Dr Keatinge coaxed. 'It's the flat one. Over there. It should be smooth.' I knew I would regret it all my life if I didn't push on. I turned left and began paralleling shore. I glanced at Dr Keatinge. He looked surprised, then worried. He must have thought I was becoming disoriented and going into hypothermia.

'Bill, it's all the way, or no way!' I shouted.

He grinned and the crew started cheering and clapping and waving their arms in the air. I rode their wave of energy, took it all in, let it carry me.

I looked at my hands pulling through the water. They looked like the purple-gray hands of a cadaver. My shoulders were blue, the colour of blueberries, and my arms, legs and trunk were splotchy white. They felt heavy, like meat taken out of a freezer. My thighs could no longer feel water being pushed past them. My face no longer felt like a face; it felt detached from my head. I started swimming faster, faster. Looking up, I could see the colours of the Soviet people's clothes, red, blue, green and black. And they were moving. They were running, slipping on the ice, picking their way down to the water's edge.

AN EPIC SWIM CAN MAKE political capital. In 1966, the Chinese paper *People's Daily* recorded that Chairman Mao, in his seventies, swam fifteen kilometres in sixty-five minutes down the Yangtze. He was supposedly propelled by the strong current, but many have queried how it could be possible to swim anywhere near that fast.

Details aside, this heroic feat proved Mao was not an old has-been who was no longer fit to rule. He had been kicked out of office after the Great Leap Forward ended in mass starvation. But after this swim, Mao was lionised by the propaganda machine controlled by his allies and was soon back in office – from where he led the Cultural Revolution.

It is true that Mao was an accomplished swimmer. Ten years earlier, in 1956, he had discovered that swimming could help him burnish his image and build his political capital. And so, he swam three of China's major rivers – the Pearl river, the Xiang and the mighty Yangtze.

After emigrating to the United States, Dr Li Zhisui, the Chairman's personal physician, wrote a biography of Mao, which was first pub-lished in 1994. Li recalls here how Mao floated alongside human waste and infectious snails, much to the consternation of his entourage who feared blame being cast upon them if any harm should come to him.

'Swimming in the Yangtze River isn't so frightening after all, is it?'
The Private Life of Chairman Mao by Dr Li Zhisui[63]

The Pearl River

Mao was showing that his determination was not to be challenged. He had begun swimming as a child, using the pond on his father's property to learn, and was a good swimmer. Now, however, everyone responsible for his safety had tried to persuade him not to swim, but the more his security staff tried to protect him, the more he insisted on swimming. He was defying us all, telling us symbolically that it was useless to attempt to restrain him.

The yacht sailed upstream a short distance and stopped as four sampans immediately surrounded it. Mao descended a ladder over the side and plunged into the water, trailed by a squadron of twenty to thirty guards, followed by the other leaders. I plunged into the water after them, joining the protective circle around Mao. Mao's decision had come so unexpectedly that he was the only one wearing a bathing suit. The rest of us were in our underwear. The river was more than a hundred yards wide, and the current was slow. The water, just as I had feared, was filthy. I saw occasional globs of human waste float by. The pollution did not bother Mao. He floated on his back, his big belly sticking up like a round balloon, legs relaxed, as though he were resting on a sofa. The water carried him downstream, and only rarely did he use his arms or legs to propel himself forward.

I was no swimmer and had to use all my energy just to stay afloat. Mao noticed my efforts and called me over to him. 'You have to relax your body,' he instructed. 'Don't move your arms and legs so much. When you want to change position, just move lightly against the water. This way you can stay in the water for a long time without so much effort. Give it a try.' I tried, but to no avail. I had to move my arms and legs or drown.

'Maybe you're afraid of sinking,' he said. 'Don't think about it. If you don't think about it, you won't sink. If you do, you will.'

We floated down the Pearl River for nearly two hours, covering some six or seven miles. Then we took showers and had lunch on board the well-equipped yacht, Mao was as elated as if he had just won a war.

'You people told me that Dr. Li said this water was too dirty,' he said to Luo Ruiqing.'

Yes,' I interjected. 'I saw human waste floating by.' Mao laughed heartily.

'If we tried to follow the standards of you physicians, we wouldn't be able to live. Don't all living things need air and water and soil? Tell me which of these things is pure? I don't believe there is any pure air, pure water, pure soil. Everything has some impurities, some dirt. If you put a fish into distilled water, how long do you think it would live?'

I was silent. Mao was clearly not going to accept my views on sanitation.

The Yangtze

Wang Renzhong had made elaborate preparations for Mao's swim. We stayed again at the East Lake guesthouse. Wang had found an elegant steamer, the *East Is Red Number One*. Mao, the leaders accompanying him, and a swelling staff that included both his own and local security personnel, boarded the boat at a factory that had been emptied of workers and filled with security guards instead. As Mao boarded the *East Is Red*, eight boats filled with security people encircled it, moving together with the steamer out to the middle of the river. Four motorboats were patrolling a still wider radius, on the lookout for anything untoward.

As the steamer reached the middle of the Yangtze, just downstream from the huge bridge that was then under construction, Mao descended the ladder and got into the water, the other leaders following. Immediately, some forty security guards formed a protective circle around the Chairman.

As I stepped from the ladder into the water, the rapid current immediately carried me some fifty yards downstream. I managed to keep my balance, floating with the water, moving my arms and legs as little as possible, trying to imitate Mao's style. The feared whirlpools were nowhere in sight, and after the initial shock I felt at the strength of the current, I was calm, floating effortlessly downstream, basking in the midday sun, as though melting into the warm brown water. The Yangtze was in flood, and from the middle of the river the banks were barely visible. It was a wonderful way to relax.

Suddenly I heard people on *The East Is Red* shouting and saw several small boats racing toward it. A number of sailors jumped into the water near the steamer. I moved closer to Mao to find out what was going on. But neither he nor anyone else knew. Only when we got back on board did we learn that three-star general Chen Zaidao, the commander of the Wuhan Military Region, had decided to enter the water alone shortly after we left. But the rapid current frightened him and he tried to swim upstream back to the boat. The powerful current overwhelmed him, and he swallowed great quantities of water. By the time the sailors reached him to haul him out, he was nearly drowned.

After about an hour of floating, Luo Ruiqing and Wang Dongxing urged me to try to convince Mao to stop. But Mao wanted to continue.

'Swimming in the Yangtze River isn't so frightening after all, is it?' he asked.

'No, not this way,' I responded.

'It seems to me,' he continued thoughtfully, 'that even the most difficult thing, the most dangerous thing, is not to be feared so long as one prepares for it well. Without good preparation, even an easy thing can create complications.' I had to agree. But he was not just talking about swimming in rivers, I suspected. His words had other implications, too.

We floated for another hour. Again, Luo and Wang urged me to get Mao back on *The East Is Red*. We were about to reach the part of the river that was heavily infested with the schistosomiasis-carrying snails. I told Mao.

'What infested area?' he demanded. 'They just want to get me back on the ship.'

'But two hours is enough,' I said. 'A lot of people didn't have a chance to eat before we started. They must be very hungry by now.'

'All right,' he agreed. 'Let's go back and eat.'

One of the sailors swimming with us estimated we had gone about fifteen miles, but I thought we had gone much further. The current was very swift. We both agreed that the swim had been effortless. We had not been exercising at all. Yang Shangkun agreed.

'This isn't swimming,' he said. 'It's just floating with a little effort.'

Once Mao was finally on board, the leaders in charge of his safety breathed a collective sigh of relief. Wang Dongxing had been particularly worried. He wondered out loud what would have happened if it had been Mao rather than Chen Zaidao who nearly drowned. 'I could have been accused of committing an unpardonable crime,' he said.

~~~~~~~~

AN EXTRAORDINARY SWIM KICKSTARTED THE legend of an acutely political man who is still, decades after he was assassinated at the age of forty-six, known by the initials JFK. With the strap of his life vest in his mouth, John F. Kennedy swam for hours to bring a wounded sailor to shore. An account of this rescue was published in *The New Yorker* magazine in 1947, and the fact that he was then regarded as a real-life hero helped to propel JFK into the presidency.

Lieutenant Kennedy was in command of patrol torpedo boat PT-109 in the Solomon Islands in 1943 when it was hit by a Japanese destroyer and broke up, with one part erupting into flames. Two sailors were killed instantly. Kennedy, who had been on the Harvard swimming team, plunged into the water and was able to drag two seriously injured men onto the part of the ship that was still afloat.

The surviving group of nine spent twelve hours clinging to the hulk, waiting for rescue. But having seen the destruction and the fire, the US Navy concluded there were no survivors and made no attempt at rescue. Eventually, Kennedy decided the men had to leave the sinking ship and make for the tiny, deserted Plum Pudding island, three and a half miles away.

Kennedy took the strap of his badly burned colleague Patrick McMahon's life vest – called a 'Mae West' – in his mouth and dragged him along for five hours, swallowing considerable amounts of water, while the rest of the crew helped two other non-swimmers along, using a timber from the ship as a flotation aid.

After reaching the rocky island and finding a few coconuts, Kennedy risked his life again by swimming to an area where he thought US boats might pass. There were none, and after treading water for an hour he tried to swim back to the others, but was swept out towards the open sea. Kennedy came very close to losing his life, but managed to grab on to a reef near the island and from there he made his way back to his men eventually, exhausted and vomiting, his bare feet bleeding from the sharp coral.

After several nights of attempts like this, Kennedy encountered some native inhabitants of the island and managed to give them a message carved in a coconut. They in turn delivered it to Reg Evans, an Australian coastwatcher who was operating from a secret base on top of the Mount Veve volcano on the island of Kolombangara. Evans rowed fifty miles to alert the US Navy and then returned to his base. The next day a native boat took Kennedy, hidden under coconut leaves, over to Evans's base. The US patrol boat picked him up there, and he guided them to the place where the men were hiding. The group were all rescued.

The coconut shell was made into a paperweight and is now on display in the JFK Presidential Library, Boston. Kennedy did not write or talk much about this episode, but in a letter to his wartime lover, the Danish journalist Inga Arvad, he reflected on his rescue of Patrick McMahon. Like many veterans of war, in this letter he dwells more on the man he didn't manage to save than on the ones he did.

'He couldn't swim and I was able to help him.'
Letter from John F. Kennedy to Inga Arvad[64]

I received a letter today from the wife of my engineer, who was so badly burnt that his face and hands were just flesh, and he was that way for six days. He couldn't swim and I was able to help him, and his wife thanked me, and in her letter she said: 'I suppose to you it was just part of your job, but Mr McMahon was part of my life and if he had died, I don't think I would have wanted to go on living.'

There are many McMahons that don't come through. There was a boy on my boat, only 24, had three kids . . . He was in the forward gun turret when the destroyer hit us.

An undated handwritten note about the period after the shipwreck and the role Reg Evans played in their rescue was found among JFK's papers when he was assassinated and it, too, is now the property of the JFK Presidential Library.

'Busy in the margin thin edge of existence.'
Handwritten note by John F. Kennedy, JFK Presidential Library[65]

I do not remember his name – I never knew it – but I'll always remember him. In late August the P.T. boat that I commanded had been cut in two, rammed and cut in two while attacking a Japanese destroyer. Then a week later the survivors, nine of us who had survived, and some were badly hurt, were busy in the margin thin edge of existence – on a narrow reef drinking rain water – eating a few odd coconuts – freezing at night – and wondering how it all would end.

About the 7th day we saw a native off the shore in a small canoe. He came in somewhat fearfully to the beach with us – he spoke no English and we carved out a message about our approximate position to on a green coconut and shouted the name of our base Rendova – Rendova and pointed east. A day later he returned in a larger war canoe with a dozen natives who built a shelter – made a fire gave us food. I rode with them for a good while – some hours away to where a New Zealander had a base – He told us that our friend had come by and told him of our troubles, and he [Evans] had left the same night to row 50 miles to our home base.

A day later a P.T. boat came to pick us up [Kennedy and Evans] . . . [After going with the PT boat to rescue the other men] he [Evans] rode back [to his base] with us. He shook hands with each of us when he got off the boat and then disappeared – back into the Jungle of Melanesia – into the islands of the Soloman. Perhaps he has forgotten all about us – but we remember him – yes – we will always remember him.

CHAPTER II

Strong Swimmers

YOU DON'T HAVE TO SWIM a long way for a swim to be epic. Here are some examples of legendary feats of endurance and skill that don't necessarily involve distance covered.

Karen Carr wrote a mould-breaking critical assessment of the history and culture of swimming, *Shifting Currents*, published in 2022. This excerpt gives context to some of the passages in this chapter; this is the misrepresentation that was going on in the background. Carr explains how the narratives invented to support slavery distorted African swimming prowess into evidence of savagery. Slavers then tried to prevent their captives from learning the art – because swimming could be a means of escape.

'Knowing how to swim divided Black from White.'
Shifting Currents: A World History of Swimming by Karen Carr[66]

Everywhere European traders arrived, they were astonished to discover that most of the people they met were excellent swimmers, better swimmers even than the best swimmers of Renaissance Europe. While even good swimmers in Europe could only use the breaststroke, Africans, Southeast Asians and Native Americans all used an overarm crawl stroke. European swimmers used a frog kick, but other people all used variants

189

of a straight-leg kick. Most could swim with their faces in the water, and many could execute elegant dives. People swam carrying children on their backs. Though some Europeans were intrigued, many of them reacted to this discovery by asserting that swimming was an activity unsuited to civilised people, appropriate only for animals and subhumans. Swimming now became racialised. Knowing how to swim divided Black from White, and the ability to swim was twisted to support the pretence that the people of Africa and the Americas were natural slaves.

This justification is not surprising, because Europeans set out for Africa precisely in search of people to enslave. The reduced crop yields of the Little Ice Age may have helped drive Europeans to explore the Atlantic Ocean, but they were not sailing to find new land to farm; they wanted new peoples to farm; they wanted saleable captives. Countries did not pay to outfit fleets of expensive ships out of an interest in science or a sense of adventure.

Europeans seized on any and all cultural differences as evidence that Africans were natural slaves. And as everything about Africans justified slavery in European slavers' eyes, so it was with Africans' ability to swim. Europeans used swimming to dehumanize Africans.

Slave traders' false suggestion that Africans swam innately, like fish, found a corollary in the idea that Africans could swim because, like animals, they were incapable of rational thought. As late as 1840, swimming books repeated this canard: 'Man cannot swim with the same faculty as many of the inferior animals, which seem to be led by instinct to use the proper action for their preservation, while rational creatures, being aware of their danger, grow fearful or impatient, and begin to struggle, which has the effect of making them sink in the water.'

New distinctions were being forged. No longer would Europeans consider swimming to be a mark of education and sophistication. Instead, Europeans now re-imagined swimming as something animals did. When people swam, Europeans took it to mean that the swimmers were practically animals themselves, and could be treated as such. Conveniently for European colonization, for the slave trade and for the European project to dominate world trade, there could be no objection to buying and selling them, renaming them, beating them or slaughtering them.

African women were just as good swimmers as the men, but their enslavers' gender prejudices often prevented these women from swimming. By the early nineteenth century enslaved African American men were also kept from learning to swim, because White slaveholders feared they would escape. Indeed, some African Americans did escape by swimming, as we know from the escape narratives of Caribbean and Brazilian maroons and the accounts of Solomon Northrup and Jacob Green, who both escaped from Southern slavery to the North. In Mark Twain's fictional *Huckleberry Finn*, similarly, the enslaved Jim swims to freedom. Swimming and water symbolised freedom and came to be a marker of African-American identity as well. But Northrup reports that enslaved African Americans were 'not allowed to learn the art of swimming' and were 'incapable of crossing the most inconsiderable stream'. Annie Davis was beaten for swimming while she was enslaved. Enslaved African Americans may also have lacked leisure to learn to swim well. Though he had fond memories of splashing in a swimming hole from his enslaved childhood, the abolitionist Frederick Douglass, for example, did not know how to swim.

~~~~~

SOLOMON NORTHRUP, WHO WAS BORN free in New York, was kidnapped and sold into slavery in the Deep South in 1841. He recovered his freedom in 1853, lectured for the Abolitionist movement and wrote his memoir, which became the bestselling *Twelve Years a Slave*, dedicated to Harriet Beecher Stowe.

In this excerpt, Northrup defends himself against a brutal attack from Tibeats, who has sub-contracted him from his owner, William Ford, to whom Northrup represents a valuable asset. Northrup overcomes Tibeats but then lets him go and flees into the swamp.

'The dogs had not gained upon me since I struck the water. Evidently they were confused.'

Twelve Years a Slave by Solomon Northrup[67]

If I killed him [Tibeats], my life must pay the forfeit—if he lived, my life only would satisfy his vengeance. A voice within whispered me to fly. To be a wanderer among the swamps, a fugitive and a vagabond on the face of the earth, was preferable to the life that I was leading.

My resolution was soon formed, and swinging him from the workbench to the ground, I leaped a fence near by, and hurried across the plantation, passing the slaves at work in the cotton field. At the end of a quarter of a mile I reached the wood-pasture, and it was a short time indeed that I had been running it. Climbing on to a high fence, I could see the cotton press, the great house, and the space between. It was a conspicuous position, from whence the whole plantation was in view. I saw Tibeats cross the field towards the house, and enter it—then he came out, carrying his saddle, and presently mounted his horse and galloped away.

I was desolate, but thankful. Thankful that my life was spared,—desolate and discouraged with the prospect before me. What would become of me? Who would befriend me? Whither should I fly? Oh, God! Thou who gavest me life, and implanted in my bosom the love of life—who filled it with emotions such as other men, thy creatures, have, do not forsake me. Have pity on the poor slave—let me not perish. If thou dost not protect me, I am lost—lost! Such supplications, silently and unuttered, ascended from my inmost heart to Heaven. But there was no answering voice—no sweet, low tone, coming down from on high, whispering to my soul, 'It is I, be not afraid.' I was the forsaken of God, it seemed—the despised and hated of men!

In about three-fourths of an hour several of the slaves shouted and made signs for me to run. Presently, looking up the bayou, I saw Tibeats and two others on horse-back, coming at a fast gait, followed by a troop of dogs. There were as many as eight or ten. Distant as I was, I knew them. They belonged on the adjoining plantation. The dogs used on Bayou Bœuf for hunting slaves are a kind of blood-hound, but a far more savage breed than is found in the Northern States. They will attack a negro, at their master's bidding, and cling to him as the common bull-dog will cling to a four footed animal. Frequently their loud bay is heard in the swamps, and then there is speculation as to what point the runaway will be overhauled—the same as a New-York hunter stops to listen to the hounds coursing along the hillsides, and suggests to his companion that the fox will be taken at such a place. I never knew a slave escaping with his life from Bayou Bœuf. One reason is, they are not allowed to learn the art of swimming, and are incapable of crossing the most inconsiderable stream. In their flight they can go in no direction but a little way without coming to a bayou, when the inevitable alternative is presented, of being drowned or overtaken by the dogs. In youth I had practised in the clear streams that flow through my native district, until I had become an expert swimmer, and felt at home in the watery element.

I stood upon the fence until the dogs had reached the cotton press.

In an instant more, their long, savage yells announced they were on my track. Leaping down from my position, I ran towards the swamp. Fear gave me strength, and I exerted it to the utmost. Every few moments I could hear the yelpings of the dogs. They were gaining upon me. Every howl was nearer and nearer. Each moment I expected they would spring upon my back—expected to feel their long teeth sinking into my flesh. There were so many of them, I knew they would tear me to pieces, that they would worry me, at once, to death. I gasped for breath—gasped forth a half-uttered, choking prayer to the Almighty to save me—to give me strength to reach some wide, deep bayou where I could throw them off the track, or sink into its waters. Presently I reached a thick palmetto bottom. As I fled through them they made a loud rustling noise, not loud enough, however, to drown the voices of the dogs.

Continuing my course due south, as nearly as I can judge, I came at length to water just over my shoe. The hounds at that moment could not have been five rods behind me. I could hear them crashing and plunging through the palmettoes, their loud, eager yells making the whole swamp clamorous with the sound. Hope revived a little as I reached the water. If it were only deeper, they might lose the scent, and thus disconcerted, afford me the opportunity of evading them. Luckily, it grew deeper the farther I proceeded—now over my ankles—now half-way to my knees—now sinking a moment to my waist, and then emerging presently into more shallow places. The dogs had not gained upon me since I struck the water. Evidently they were confused. Now their savage intonations grew more and more distant, assuring me that I was leaving them. Finally I stopped to listen, but the long howl came booming on the air again, telling me I was not yet safe. From bog to bog, where I had stepped, they could still keep upon the track, though impeded by the water. At length, to my great joy, I came to a wide bayou, and plunging in, had soon stemmed its sluggish current to the other side. There, certainly, the dogs would be confounded—the current carrying down the stream all traces of that slight, mysterious scent, which enables the quick-smelling hound to follow in the track of the fugitive.

After crossing this bayou the water became so deep I could not run. I was now in what I afterwards learned was the 'Great Pacoudrie Swamp'. It was filled with immense trees—the sycamore, the gum, the cotton wood and cypress, and extends, I am informed, to the shore of the Calcasieu river. For thirty or forty miles it is without inhabitants, save wild beasts—the bear, the wild-cat, the tiger, and great slimy reptiles, that are crawling through it everywhere. Long before I reached the bayou, in fact, from the time I struck the water until I emerged from the swamp on my return, these reptiles surrounded me. I saw hundreds of moccasin snakes. Every log and bog—every trunk of a fallen tree, over which I was compelled to step or climb, was alive with them. They crawled away at my approach, but sometimes in my haste, I almost placed my hand or foot upon them. They are poisonous serpents—their bite more fatal than the rattlesnake's. Besides, I had lost one shoe, the sole having come entirely off, leaving the upper only dangling to my ankle.

I saw also many alligators, great and small, lying in the water, or on pieces of floodwood. The noise I made usually startled them, when they moved off and plunged into the deepest places. Sometimes, however, I would come directly upon a monster before observing it. In such cases, I would start back, run a short way round, and in that manner shun them. Straight forward, they will run a short distance rapidly, but do not possess the power of turning. In a crooked race, there is no difficulty in evading them.

About two o'clock in the afternoon, I heard the last of the hounds. Probably they did not cross the bayou. Wet and weary, but relieved from the sense of instant peril, I continued on, more cautious and afraid, however, of the snakes and alligators than I had been in the earlier portion of my flight. Now, before stepping into a muddy pool, I would strike the water with a stick. If the waters moved, I would go around it, if not, would venture through.

At length the sun went down, and gradually night's trailing mantle shrouded the great swamp in darkness. Still I staggered on, fearing every instant I should feel the dreadful sting of the moccasin, or be crushed within the jaws of some disturbed alligator. The dread of them now almost equaled the fear of the pursuing hounds. The moon arose after a time, its mild light creeping through the overspreading branches, loaded with long, pendent moss. I kept traveling forwards until after midnight, hoping all the while that I would soon emerge into some less desolate and dangerous region. But the water grew deeper and the walking more difficult than ever. I perceived it would be impossible to proceed much farther, and knew not, moreover, what hands I might fall into, should I succeed in reaching a human habitation. Not provided with a pass, any white man would be at liberty to arrest me, and place me in prison until such time as my master should 'prove property, pay charges, and take me away.' I was an estray, and if so unfortunate as to meet a law-abiding citizen of Louisiana, he would deem it his duty to his neighbor, perhaps, to put me forthwith in the pound. Really, it was difficult to determine which I had most reason to fear—dogs, alligators or men!

After midnight, however, I came to a halt. Imagination cannot picture the dreariness of the scene. The swamp was resonant with the quacking of innumerable ducks! Since the foundation of the earth, in all probability, a human footstep had never before so far penetrated the recesses of the swamp. It was not silent now—silent to a degree that rendered it oppressive,—as it was when the sun was shining in the heavens. My midnight intrusion had awakened the feathered tribes, which seemed to throng the morass in hundreds of thousands, and their garrulous throats poured forth such multitudinous sounds—there was such a fluttering of wings—such sullen plunges in the water all around me—that I was affrighted and appalled. All the fowls of the air, and all the creeping things of the earth appeared to have assembled together in that particular place, for the purpose of filling it with clamor and confusion. Not by human dwellings—not in crowded cities alone, are the sights and sounds of life. The wildest places of the earth are full of them. Even in the heart of that dismal swamp, God had provided a refuge and a dwelling place for millions of living things.

The moon had now risen above the trees, when I resolved upon a new project. Thus far I had endeavored to travel as nearly south as possible. Turning about I proceeded in a north-west direction, my object being to strike the Pine Woods in the vicinity of Master Ford's. Once within the shadow of his protection, I felt I would be comparatively safe.

My clothes were in tatters, my hands, face, and body covered with scratches, received from the sharp knots of fallen trees, and in climbing over piles of brush and floodwood. My bare foot was full of thorns. I was besmeared with muck and mud, and the green slime that had collected on the surface of the dead water, in which I had been immersed to the neck many times during the day and night. Hour after hour, and tiresome indeed had they become, I continued to plod along on my north-west course. The water began to grow less deep, and the ground more firm under my feet. At last I reached the Pacoudrie, the same wide bayou I had swam while 'outward bound.' I swam it again, and shortly after thought I heard a cock crow, but the sound was faint, and it might have been a mockery of the ear. The water receded from my advancing footsteps—now I had left the bogs behind me—now I was on dry land that gradually ascended to the plain, and I knew I was somewhere in the 'Great Pine Woods'.

Just at day-break I came to an opening—a sort of small planta-tion—but one I had never seen before. In the edge of the woods I came upon two men, a slave and his young master, engaged in catching wild hogs. The white man I knew would demand my pass, and not able to give him one, would take me into possession. I was too wearied to run again, and too desperate to be taken, and therefore adopted a ruse that proved entirely successful. Assuming a fierce expression, I walked directly towards him, looking him steadily in the face. As I approached, he moved backwards with an air of alarm. It was plain he was much affrighted—that he looked upon me as some infernal goblin, just arisen from the bowels of the swamp!

'Where does William Ford live?' I demanded, in no gentle tone.

'He lives seven miles from here,' was the reply.

'Which is the way to his place?' I again demanded, trying to look more fiercely than ever.

'Do you see those pine trees yonder?' he asked, pointing to two, a mile distant, that rose far above their fellows, like a couple of tall sentinels, overlooking the broad expanse of forest.

'I see them,' was the answer.

'At the feet of those pine trees,' he continued, 'runs the Texas road. Turn to the left, and it will lead you to William Ford's.'

~~~

IN 1696 IN PARIS, THE publisher Charles Moette printed *The Art of Swimming* by scientist and traveller Melchisédech Thévenot (this was the book that taught Benjamin Franklin to swim). Thévenot's influential book noted that – contrary to what was later claimed – swimming prowess was common in the world beyond Europe among non-Caucasian peoples.

'It is most certain that the Indians and the Blacks excel all others in their arts of swimming and diving.'

The Art of Swimming by Melchisédech Thévenot[68]

Both Grecian and Roman histories are full of narratives of the undertakings of divers. But to come to our times it is most certain that the Indians and the Blacks excel all others in their arts of swimming and diving. Tis to them the ladies are obliged for their ornaments of pearls. They are the divers who fish for them. They are also very useful in recovering anchors and merchandise that has been cast away.

The Chinese are not much inferior to them in this sort of exercise. They extremely apply themselves to it. They have whole floating towns which they build upon reeds and the houses are joined together, with all other appurtenances of towns upon land.

~

THERE ARE FEW WRITTEN ACCOUNTS of women swmming outside Europe, but one is from Ibn Battuta. The fourteenth-century Maghrebi traveller, explorer and scholar frequently mentions the slave girls he bought and sold as he crossed Africa and Asia in the memoir he dictated, commonly known as *The Rihla*. Here, he recalls how he survived a shipwreck and how one of the slave girls he has acquired demonstrates her prowess at swimming. It is just as well she could swim – as Batutta's favourite is the one who gets the place on the life raft.

'The other girl said: I am a good swimmer.'
A Gift to Those Who Contemplate the Wonders of Cities and the Marvels of Travelling by Ibn Battuta[69]

During the voyage a gale sprang up and our ship nearly took in water. We had no knowledgeable pilot on board. We came to some rocks on which the ship narrowly escaped being wrecked, and then into some shallows where the ship ran aground. We were face to face with death, and people jettisoned all that they had, and bade farewell to one another. We cut down the mast and threw it overboard, and the sailors made a wooden raft. We were then about two farsakhs from the shore. I was going to climb down to the raft, when my companions (for I had two slave-girls and two of my companions with me) said to me: Are you going to go down and leave us? So I put their safety before my own and said: You two go down and take with you the girl that I love.' The other girl said: I am a good swimmer and I shall hold on to one of the raft ropes and swim with them.'

So both my companions (the one being Muhammad b. Farhān al-Tūzari, and the other an Egyptian) and the one girl went on the raft, the other girl swimming. The sailors tied ropes to the raft, and swam with their aid. I sent along with them all the things that I valued and the gems and ambergris, and they reached the shore in safety because the wind was in their favour. I myself stayed on the ship.

The captain made his way ashore on the rudder. The sailors set to work to make four rafts, but night fell before they were completed, and the ship took in water. I climbed on the poop and stayed there until morning, when a party of infidels came out to us in a boat and we went ashore with them to the coast of Ma'bar. We told them that we were friends of their Sultan, under whose protection they live, and they wrote informing him of this. He was then two days journey away, on an expedition, and I too wrote to him telling him what had happened to me.

Those infidels took us into a great jungle and brought us some fruit resembling melons. This is produced by the muql tree and has inside it what resembles cotton containing a honey-like substance which they extract and from which they make a sweet called by them tall, resembling sugar. They brought also some good fish. We stayed there three days at the end of which an amir called Qamar al-Din arrived from the Sultan with a body of horse and foot, bringing a palanquin and ten horses.

~

THERE ARE MANY ANCIENT TEXTS in Japanese literature about the theory and practice of Samurai and Ninja swimming, but they are not often available in English. In her personal exploration from 2021, Japanese American writer Bonnie Tsui dives into the practice and gives us a flavour of this incredible art.

'The armor is very heavy . . . But I'm delighted I can swim.'
Why We Swim by Bonnie Tsui[70]

When I find out that there are Samurai swimming competitions being held today in Japan – now picture that silent samurai gliding across a 25-meter swimming pool – that attract swimmers from as far away as

Poland and England, I make the trip to Tokyo to seek out the leading practitioners of Nibon eibo.

In a Japanese television report, a samurai lowers himself into a swimming pool. I watch closely as he demonstrates katchu gozen oyogi, tull armor swimming. He moves smoothly on a sideways path across the pool, legs alternately circling, the metal-pronged helmet on his head stays dry. Despite the blanket of riveted leather scales weighing down his torso, les slides along, wraithlike.

'The armor is very heavy,' he says with a little smile, after he has dragged himself out of the pool. 'But I'm delighted I can swim.'

Another swimmer, this one dressed in swimming trunks and a black cap with white stripes, demonstrates a different position, the swimmer surges vertically out of the water, arms whipping back and head thrust forward, exposed to his very lean (and very tan) waist. It is the fundamental method of jumping while swimming to disentangle oneself from seaweed or other debris, or to leap onto a boat.

Finally, the most fundamental of all moves: tachi-oyogi, standing swimming. The young competitor's face is relaxed, his eyes trained on the horizon. His head moves near imperceptibly, the water in front of him as still as glass. It's as if he is on a very slow treadmill hidden just below the surface of the water. His head and hair are completely dry. Different schools have different variations, but the basics are the same. That familiar egg-beater kick used today by synchronised Swimmers and water-polo players to propel their upper bodies so powerfully out of the water? It bears a strong resemblance to the method described in detail in sixteenth-century master scrolls from the Kobori ryu which specializes in techniques to free up the hands. The muted cycling of the legs is meant to be efficient and to keep the upper body stationary and stable. The version of the egg-beater kick used by the Japanese synchronised swimming team comes directly from the Nojima ryu.

I learn that if you're good at standing swimming, you can do anything in the water: write calligraphy, load and fire a rifle, duel with swords. You can carry weapons and flags. You can shoot a bow and arrow with great accuracy while nearly submerged. Remember that the feathers on an arrow need to be dry to fly true.

In the news segment, we see two men fight, each gripping his wooden sword with both hands. They shout and circle each other warily, as if they are dancing. But they're treading water, in a lake, far from shore. We see two women swimming nukite, the withdrawing hand style. This high-elbow, crawling arm technique is used to swim facing the wind and waves or when crossing the tide; it allows you to cut through the waves with your shoulder and avoid being overwhelmed by the foamy force of a breaking wave.

Midori Ishibiki is a modern-day master in the age-old art of samurai swimming. Appointed by the Japan Swimming Federation, Midori is one of eight people who are responsible for preserving the swimming martial art of Japan. Like any other martial art – judo, say, or kendo – Nihon eihe is governed by various levels of practice, and each level requires years of training and exams to move up to the next.

Midori grew up in Tokyo and now lives in Kamakura, a seaside town an hour south of the city. Fifty years old, with stylish brown hair styled in a bob framing her round face, she can glide across a pool with barely a ripple. But Nibon eibo isn't just about physical skills: 'It also emphasizes a spiritual path,' she says in her perky British-accented English, which comes from years of living in Norwich. 'It's like meditation.'

Old Japanese texts teach that swimming in freezing water cultivates perseverance; submergence leads to patience; diving fosters bravery. Floating of the body leads to serenity of the mind. The mastery of rescue and resuscitation is a sign of wholehearted benevolence.

Midori began studying classical swimming techniques with her master when she was thirteen, during summers at the beach in Chiba, across Tokyo Bay from the city of Tokyo. Her club's current master, Kazuo Yamaguchi, is now in his mid-eighties, and Midori still studies with him every summer. But these days the student is also a master, and while in Chiba she in turn instructs more than two hundred junior high students from their school's clubhouse. Theirs is the Suitu ryu, which devised practical ways to swim efficiently on the open sea and rivers – to safely get through waves, say, or to quickly retrieve something floating nearby. Though samurai swimming is at the roots of Japan's swimming culture, its traditions are waning. But those tasked with its preservation see a direct line to modern Japanese swimming success in international competition. During an unseasonably balmy week in early May, I travel around Tokyo to see what samurai swimming looks like today and what it means that people are still doing it.

My pursuit of Midori Ishibiki leads me to an indoor swimming club in Yokohama, where I am sweating profusely on the pool deck. The indoor pool deck is like a sauna turned up to the max. It causes me distress to be dressed in sweat clothes by the edge of a perfectly nice pool, but it's the only way I can take proper notes on the happenings in Midori's swim class. Today there are five Hanshi masters – the highest level master there is in Nibon attending the class along with the regular students. One of the masters, Masaki Imamura, the seventy-three-year-old vice chair of the Japan Swimming Federation's committee on Nibon eibo, is examining me curiously. He also thinks it's weird that I'm wearing street clothes.

'Why don't you swim?' he greets me with a deep, booming voice, as he issues forth a charming grin. 'It is very hot.' He is wearing a black

Speedo and a black cloth swim cap with white piping and strings that tie under his chin. The black cap indicates seniority in the Shinden ryu; white caps are given to beginners, much like the white belt in other martial arts like judo or karate. The progression of colours, however, varies by ryu. I manage to smile back, then grimace, and I'm tempted to dash back into the locker room to shed my heavy cotton dress and leggings so I can get in that water, too. But I can't chance missing what happens next.

The fifteen men and women in Midori's class circle and bow. Then, one by one, they stride to the water and slip in, smoothly and soundlessly, like ducks to the surface of a lake. Imamura hops out and volunteers to be my de facto sports announcer. 'Why do we swim?' rumbles Imamura, with another winning smile. 'Well, that's very simple, you see.' Like a professor, he steeples his hands and proceeds to tick off the following on his slender brown fingers:

For survival: 'Japan, of course, is surrounded by water.'

For religion: 'In Shinto practices, misogi-the ritualistic cleaning of body and mind with water is sacred.'

For fighting: 'The samurai, to protect feudal territory, developed regionally specific swimming schools.'

For competition: 'Disciplines include diving and racing, say, or synchronised swimming.'

For strength of mind and body: 'The topmost principle in Nibon eibo is mind and water, together.'

This last principle, he says, can be explained as Mizu no Kokoro, or 'mind like water.' On the bench next to us, he traces a finger on its surface with water as he speaks, writing out the Japanese characters. 'This is the most important thing. There are many reasons, but when you get older, you appreciate the Zen part, the master part, the philosophy.'

CHAPTER III

Ancients

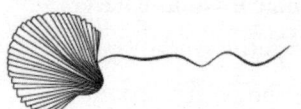

THE ANCIENT GREEKS REGARDED SWIMMING as part of an elementary education and many legendary heroes were swimmers, most especially Odysseus. *The Odyssey* has a special resonance for me as, when I was at school, an ambitious drama teacher turned it into a play for our summer show. My line – borrowed from Tennyson's 'The Lotus Eaters' was: '"Courage!" said one and pointed to the land. "A mounting wave shall roll us shoreward soon."' The only other thing I remember is a hapless cast member, who had to say: 'The cows! They're coming alive!' and step backwards, falling off the stage on the opening night.

In this excerpt, the sea god Poseidon has caused a storm which has shipwrecked our hero as he escapes from Calypso's enchanted isle on a raft. Athena intervenes to calm the waves and Odysseus manages to swim to Scheria (Corfu). Incidentally, Odysseus's technique here of grabbing onto a rock to avoid being thrown against it by the tide is also used in the book by Daniel Defoe where Robinson Crusoe survives shipwreck in a similar style.

'He heard the boom of the sea upon the reefs.'

The Odyssey by Homer[71]

Then for two nights and two days he was driven about over the swollen waves, and full-often his heart foreboded destruction. But when fair-tressed Dawn brought to its birth the third day, then the wind ceased and there was a windless calm, and he caught sight of the shore close at hand.

Odysseus swam on, eager to set foot on the land. But when he was as far away as a man's voice carries when he shouts, he heard the boom of the sea upon the reefs—for the great waves thundered against the dry land, belching upon it in terrible fashion.

While he pondered, a great wave bore him against the rugged shore. There would his skin have been stripped off and his bones broken, had not the goddess, flashing-eyed Athena, put a thought in his mind. On he rushed and seized the rock with both hands, and clung to it, groaning, until the great wave went by. Thus then did he escape this wave, but in its backward flow it once more rushed upon him and smote him, and flung him far out in the sea. And just as, when a cuttlefish is dragged from its hole, many pebbles cling to its suckers, even so from his strong hands were bits of skin stripped off against the rocks; and the great wave covered him. Then verily would hapless Odysseus have perished beyond his fate, had not flashing-eyed Athena given him prudence.

Making his way forth from the surge where it belched upon the shore, he swam outside, looking ever toward the land in hope to find shelving beaches and harbors of the sea. But when, as he swam, he came to the mouth of a fair-flowing river, where seemed to him the best place, since it was smooth of stones, and besides there was shelter from the wind, he knew the river as he flowed forth, and prayed to Poseidon in his heart.

The god straightway stayed his stream, and checked the waves, and made a calm before him, and brought him safely to the mouth of the river.

~

POSEIDON IS A FEARSOME ENTITY and he definitely has it in for Odysseus, constantly throwing obstacles in the way of even the simplest journey. The early nineteenth-century poet Heinrich Heine, a sharply witty and critical German Jew, portrays him as a coarse bully. Here, the narrator is safe to travel by sea only because of his complete lack of importance.

'So spake Poseidon, and sank him again in the sea.'
'Poseidon' from *North Sea Song* by Heinrich Heine[72]

Alone on the strand, I read the song of Odysseus,
Sighing I spoke: "Thou evil Poseidon,
Thy wrath is fearful, and I myself dread
For my own voyage homeward."
The words were scarce spoken,
When up foamed the sea,
And from the sparkling waters rose he,
The mighty bulrush-crowned sea god,
And scornfully cried: — "Be not afraid, little poet
I will not in endanger thy wretched vessel,
Nor rock thy being with terrible shaking.
"For thou, little poet, hast not troubled me,
Thou hast not damaged even a chimney pot
In the great sacred palace of Priam,

Nor even an eyelash hast thou singed,
In the eye of my son Polyphemus;
Nor did you protect the goddess of wisdom,
Pallas Athene from my wrath."
So spake Poseidon, and sank him again in the sea
And over the vulgar sailor's joke,
Laughed under the water Amphitrite, the fat old fish-wife,
And the stupid daughters of Nereus.

~~~

THE ANCIENT ROMANS COULD SWIM too – the women as well as the men. The Roman maiden Cloelia was taken hostage as part of a peace deal between the city-state of Rome and the Etruscans in around 500 BCE. King Posena's army had laid siege to Rome for many months, and food was growing scarce, when the city handed over captives as part of the deal. In his *The History of Rome*, Livy, writing in the first century BCE, tells the story of her heroic escape.

'This action surpassed those of Cocles and Mucius.'
'Conduct of Cloelia', *The History of Rome* by Livy[73]

As the camp of the Etrurians had been pitched not far from the banks of the Tiber, a young woman named Cloelia, one of the hostages, deceiving her guards, swam over the river, amidst the arrows of the enemy, at the head of a troop of maidens, and brought them all safe to their families.

When the king was informed of this, at first highly incensed, he sent deputies to Rome to demand the hostage Cloelia; saying that he did not regard the others. Afterwards, being changed into admiration of her courage, he said, 'that this action surpassed those of Cocles and Mucius,' and declared, 'as he would consider the treaty as broken if the hostage were not delivered up, so, if given up, he would send her back safe to her friends.'

Both sides kept their faith: the Romans restored their pledge of peace according to treaty; and with the king of Etruria merit found not only security, but honour; and, after making encomiums on the young lady, promised to give her, as a present, half of the hostages, and that she should choose whom she pleased.

When they were all brought out, she is said to have pitched upon the young boys below puberty, which was both consonant to maiden delicacy, and by consent of the hostages themselves, it was deemed reasonable, that that age which was most exposed to injury should be freed from the enemy's hand.

The peace being re-established, the Romans marked the uncommon instance of bravery in the woman by an uncommon kind of honour, an equestrian statue; the statue representing a lady sitting on horseback was placed at the top of the Via Sacra.

<hr />

WHEN EUROPEANS STARTED TO REDISCOVER swimming, they linked it to the heroes of the ancient world, from whose texts they also borrowed many of their justifications for imperialism. Britain's military leaders were bred on stories of these ancient heroes. The Duke of Wellington claimed that the battle of Waterloo was 'won on the playing fields of Eton'. The culture of such schools was centred on a deep admiration of sporting prowess in athletics, in team sports and in the frigid waters of the pool or pond. Wellington could equally have spot-lighted 'the swimming pools of Harrow' as a source of military victory.

Winston Churchill, who represented his house in swimming com-petitions when at Harrow – and, as seaside photos of him in a swimsuit in the 1920s show, enjoyed bathing throughout his life – won a prize for committing to memory *The Lays of Ancient Rome*. This collection of pastiche Roman ballad verse by Thomas Barrington Macaulay, a colonial-era lawyer and civil servant, was first published in 1842. The martial speech he put into Horatius's mouth is often quoted in movies about Winston Churchill – but it is of course a piece of Victorian inven-tion rather than an original Roman text. Macaulay embellishes the tale told by Livy in a couple of paragraphs in his *The History of Rome* – he did not do the same for Cloelia, or she might be better known today.

'Oh, Tiber! Father Tiber! To whom the Romans pray.' 'A Lay Made About the Year of the City CCCLX.'

The Lays of Ancient Rome by Thomas Barrington Macaulay[74]

Then out spake brave Horatius,
The Captain of the Gate:
'To every man upon this earth
Death cometh soon or late.
And how can man die better
Than facing fearful odds,
For the ashes of his fathers,
And the temples of his Gods'.

In the story, Horatius, with two companions, holds the narrow en-trance to the only bridge across the Tiber against an approaching

Etruscan army. Standing at the head of the bridge, the trio challenges the invaders to single combat. This gives the Roman engineers time to demolish the bridge – thus preventing the invading army from rushing on the unprepared city. While his two comrades run back across the bridge just before it falls, Horatius is left stranded on the wrong side of the river.

Alone stood brave Horatius,
But constant still in mind;
Thrice thirty thousand foes before,
And the broad flood behind . . .
And he spake to the noble river
That rolls by the towers of Rome.
'Oh, Tiber! Father Tiber!
To whom the Romans pray,
A Roman's life, a Roman's arms,
Take thou in charge this day!'
So he spake, and speaking sheathed
The good sword by his side,
And with his harness on his back,
Plunged headlong in the tide.
No sound of joy or sorrow
Was heard from either bank;
But friends and foes in dumb surprise,
With parted lips and straining eyes,
Stood gazing where he sank;
And when above the surges,
They saw his crest appear,
All Rome sent forth a rapturous cry.

CHAPTER IV

Alongside Swim Heroes

SWIM ENOUGH AND SOMEONE WILL quote a line from Lord Byron's ironic epic – 'he was drown'd, and I've the ague'. Byron recreated the Greek hero Leander's swim across the Hellespont to be with his lover Hero, but it was the verse he wrote that began a trend.

Every night Leander would swim the Hellespont to make love to Hero. Each night, Hero lit a lamp in the tower which would act as a lighthouse. But on one stormy night, the flame in the lamp blew out. Leander lost sight of the shore and, lost in the storm, he drowned.

The style of the poem is mock epic, but Byron's achievement of swimming the Hellespont was genuine and impressive – and all the more so because he achieved the full swim not using a triathlete's crawl (which hadn't yet been 'invented'), but a strong breaststroke – the same stroke as used by Captain Webb in his 1875 Channel crossing. Byron failed on his first attempt, but tried again.

Byron, a direct descendant of Scotland's Stuart kings, spent his early childhood with his mother in Aberdeenshire, where he learned to swim in the Dee and Don rivers. He had a club foot (congenital talipes equinovarus) and found that in the water he was able to equal and surpass the athletic feats of his companions. He also used open water swimming to manage his mental health, taking to the water when he felt emotionally overwhelmed or in a low mood.

Many of Byron's swimming feats are recounted in Charles Sprawson's *Haunts of the Black Masseur*, including an instance where on leaving a palazzo in Venice, rather than taking a gondola, Byron flung himself fully clothed into the water and swam back to his lodgings.

'This morning I swam from Sestos to Abydos,' wrote Lord Byron in a letter to his friend, Henry Drury, on 3 May 1810. 'The immediate distance is not above a mile but the current renders it hazardous, so much so, that I doubt whether Leander's conjugal powers must not have been exhausted in his passage to Paradise.'

'To cross thy stream, broad Hellespont!'

Written After Swimming from Sestos to Abydos by Lord Byron[75]

> If, in the month of dark December,
> Leander, who was nightly wont
> (What maid will not the tale remember?)
> To cross thy stream, broad Hellespont!
> If, when the wintry tempest roar'd,
> He sped to Hero, nothing loth,
> And thus of old thy current pour'd,
> Fair Venus! how I pity both!
> For me, degenerate modern wretch,
> Though in the genial month of May,
> My dripping limbs I faintly stretch,
> And think I've done a feat today.
> But since he cross'd the rapid tide,
> According to the doubtful story,
> To woo, and Lord knows what beside,

And swam for Love, as I for Glory;
'Twere hard to say who fared the best:
Sad mortals! thus the gods still plague you!
He lost his labour, I my jest;
For he was drown'd, and I've the ague.

~~~

THE EARLY TWENTIETH-CENTURY ENGLISH POET A. E. Housman
takes the same subject here. This poem focuses on the moment when
Leander, lying in bed with Hero, contemplates his homeward journey.

'The seas he swam from earth to earth.'

'Tarry, delight, so seldom met' by A. E. Housman[76]

Tarry, delight, so seldom met,
So sure to perish, tarry still;
Forbear to cease or languish yet,
Though soon you must and will.
By Sestos town, in Hero's tower,
On Hero's heart Leander lies;
The signal torch has burned its hour
And sputters as it dies.
Beneath him, in the nighted firth,
Between two continents complain
The seas he swam from earth to earth
And he must swim again.

~~~

THE STORY OF HERO AND Leander has parallels in New Zealand's Hinemoa and Tūtāneka, although here the genders are reversed and it is the woman who makes the epic swim to be reunited with her lover. Her feat is emulated annually by hundreds of people each year in the open water Hinemoa Swim – a rare event in which the intricately carved trophy for the winning woman is bigger and more impressive than that for the victorious man.

Hinemoa was forbidden to travel by canoe from the shores of Lake Rotorua to marry her lover, who lived on the sacred island of Mokoia. So she swam the three kilometres, guided by his flute-playing, using reeds to help herself stay afloat. This story has a happy ending. Hinemoa made it and the family relented and allowed them to marry.

The song below, based on lyrics sung by Māori soldiers in the First World War and first published in 1919, is the song Tūtāneka uses to guide his love towards him.

'They are agitated, the waters of Waiapu.'
Pōkarekare Ana[77]

> They are agitated,
> the waters of Waiapu,
> But when you cross over girl,
> they will be calm.
>
> Oh girl,
> return to me,
> I could die
> of love for you.

I have written my letter,
I have sent my ring,
so that your people can see
that I am troubled.

My poor pen is shattered,
I have no more paper,
But my love
is still steadfast.

My love will never
be dried by the sun,
it will be forever moistened
by my tears.

~~~

ANOTHER EPIC SWIM THAT IS recreated annually by thousands of people, in the biggest open water swim in Europe, is that of Edmond Dantès which inspired the Défi de Monte Cristo.

French novelist Alexandre Dumas was the grandson of an African slave, Marie-Cesette Dumas, who lived on a plantation in Haiti. Alexandre wrote one of his two most enduringly popular tales, *The Count of Monte Cristo*, completed in 1844, as a serial (the other was *The Three Musketeers*).

The novel's hero Edmond Dantès ends up falsely imprisoned on a rocky island in the bay of Marseilles, about 3.5 kilometres from the city. It really was used as a prison in the nineteenth century, like Alcatraz off the coast of San Francisco, and its heavily fortified ruin is still visible today. It's Dumas's book that made it famous.

In the story, Dantès' elderly mentor, Abbe Faria, dies and his body is put in a sack. Dantès uses a tunnel between their two cells to switch places with Faria and hide himself in the sack, expecting to dig himself out of a shallow grave. But instead, a cannonball is tied to his legs and he is thrown into the sea.

'He found with pleasure that his captivity had taken away nothing of his power.'
The Count of Monte Cristo by Alexandre Dumas[78]

Dantès, although stunned and almost suffocated, had sufficient presence of mind to hold his breath, and as his right hand (prepared as he was for every chance) held his knife open, he rapidly ripped up the sack, extricated his arm, and then his body; but in spite of all his efforts to free himself from the shot, he felt it dragging him down still lower. He then bent his body, and by a desperate effort severed the cord that bound his legs, at the moment when it seemed as if he were actually strangled. With a mighty leap he rose to the surface of the sea, while the shot dragged down to the depths the sack that had so nearly become his shroud.

Dantès waited only to get breath, and then dived, to avoid being seen. When he arose a second time, he was fifty paces from where he had first sunk. He saw overhead a black and tempestuous sky, across which the wind was driving clouds that occasionally suffered a twinkling star to appear; before him was the vast expanse of waters, sombre and terrible, whose waves foamed and roared as if before the approach of a storm. Behind him, blacker than the sea, blacker than the sky, rose phantom-like the vast stone structure, whose projecting crags seemed like arms extended to seize their prey, and on the highest rock was a torch lighting two figures.

He fancied that these two forms were looking at the sea; doubtless, these strange grave-diggers had heard his cry. Dantès dived again, and remained a long time beneath the water. This was an easy feat to him, for he usually attracted a crowd of spectators in the bay before the light-house at Marseilles when he swam there, and was unanimously declared to be the best swimmer in the port. When he came up again the light had disappeared.

He must now get his bearings. Often in prison, Faria had said to him, when he saw him idle and inactive:

'Dantès, you must not give way to this listlessness; you will be drowned if you seek to escape, and your strength has not been properly exercised and prepared for exertion.'

These words rang in Dantès' ears, even beneath the waves; he hastened to cleave his way through them to see if he had not lost his strength. He found with pleasure that his captivity had taken away nothing of his power, and that he was still master of that element on whose bosom he had so often sported as a boy.

CHAPTER V

Lost

SOME HEROES DON'T MAKE IT. Certain swims are remembered in the history books because an important person lost their life. In other cases, the quality of writing gives literary immortality to someone who might otherwise have been forgotten.

Historians disagree as to whether the 68-year-old Holy Roman Emperor Frederick Barbarossa drowned or suffered a heart attack while swimming. But they agree that Barbarossa's unexpected death in a river in 1190 was a major factor in the splintering of the allied forces under his command and in the defeat of the Third Crusade.

This contemporaneous account suggests that the great leader wanted to avoid climbing a steep mountain in extreme heat and so decided to swim across what seemed like a fairly insignificant stream instead.

'Thou shalt not swim against the river's current.'
Historia de Expeditione Frederici Imperatoris[79]

On June 10 the advance unit of the army camped on the plains of Seleucea. Up to this point the whole army of the Holy Cross – the rich and the poor, the sick and those who seemed healthy had journeyed through the glare of the sun and the burning heat of summer along a tortuous road which led them across rocky cliffs accessible only to birds and mountain goats.

The Emperor, who had shared in all the dangers, wished both to moderate the inordinate heat and to avoid climbing the mountain peak. Accordingly, he attempted to swim across the very swift Calycadmus River. As the wise man says, however, 'Thou shalt not swim against the river's current.' [Eccles. 4:32]

Wise though he was in other ways, the Emperor foolishly tried his strength against the current and power of the river. Although everyone tried to stop him, he entered the water and plunged into a whirlpool. He, who had often escaped great dangers, perished miserably. Let us comment the secret judgment of God, 'to Whom no man dares say: Why have you acted thus,' when he takes such or so many men in death . . . When, therefore, the other nobles around him hastened, although too late, to help him, they took him from the water and dragged him to the bank.

Everyone was afflicted with great sorrow over his death; so much so, indeed, that some, caught between hope and dread, would have ended their lives with him. Others, however, despaired and, as it seemed that God did not care for them, they renounced the Christian faith to become pagans among the heathen.

Mourning and unrestrained sorrow – not unmerited by the death of such a prince – occupied the hearts of all, so that they could rightly lament, saying with the prophet: 'Alas, we are sinners, the wreath has faded from our brows; there are sad hearts everywhere.'

JOHN MILTON WROTE HIS POEM 'Lycidas' to commemorate his friend and classmate, Edward King, a scholar who planned to enter the Church of England, but who, in August 1637, was shipwrecked and drowned in the Irish Sea on his way to visit his family. Milton recasts Edward as the shepherd Lycidas, in a pastoral elegy which contains reflections on the meaning of life and the purpose of poetry.

'Weep no more, woeful shepherds, weep no more.'
'Lycidas' by John Milton[80]

> Weep no more, woeful shepherds, weep no more,
> For Lycidas, your sorrow, is not dead,
> Sunk though he be beneath the wat'ry floor;
> So sinks the day-star in the ocean bed,
> And yet anon repairs his drooping head,
> And tricks his beams, and with new spangled ore
> Flames in the forehead of the morning sky:
> So Lycidas sunk low, but mounted high
> Through the dear might of him that walk'd the waves
> Where, other groves and other streams along,
> With nectar pure his oozy locks he laves,
> And hears the unexpressive nuptial song,
> In the blest kingdoms meek of joy and love.

~

THE POET PERCY SHELLEY WAS fascinated by water but he was unable to learn to swim. He often predicted that he would drown at sea, and his eventual death aged only twenty-nine after a couple of close shaves lends poignancy to the poems that seemed to prefigure this fate. Shelley's wife Mary, the celebrated author of *Frankenstein*, recounted the circumstances of her husband's tragic accident in a preface to an edition of his poems.

'The sea roared unremittingly, so that we almost fancied ourselves on board ship.'
Note on Poems of 1822 by Mrs. Shelley[81]

The winter of 1822 was passed in Pisa . . . Spring sprang up early, and with extreme beauty. Shelley's passion for boating was fostered at this time by having among our friends several sailors. His favourite companion, Edward Ellerker Williams, of the 8th Light Dragoons, had begun his life in the navy, and his love for adventure and manly exercises accorded with Shelley's taste. It was their favourite plan to build a boat such as they could manage themselves. Captain Roberts, R.N., undertook to build the boat at Genoa, where he was also occupied in building the 'Bolivar' for Lord Byron. Ours was to be an open boat, on a model taken from one of the royal dockyards. I have since heard that there was a defect in this model, and that it was never seaworthy.

In the month of February, Shelley and his friend went to Spezia to seek for houses for us. Only one was to be found at all suitable; however, a trifle such as not finding a house could not stop Shelley; the one found was to serve for all. It was unfurnished; we sent our furniture by sea, and with a good deal of precipitation, arising from his impatience, made our removal. We left Pisa on the 26th of April.

The Bay of Spezia is of considerable extent, and divided by a rocky promontory into a larger and smaller one. The town of Lerici is situated on the eastern point, and in the depth of the smaller bay, which bears the name of this town, is the village of San Terenzo. Our house, Casa Magni, was close to this village; the sea came up to the door, a steep hill sheltered it behind . . . The scene was of unimaginable beauty. The blue extent of waters, the almost landlocked bay, the near castle of Lerici shutting it in to the east, and distant Porto Venere to the west; the varied forms of the precipitous rocks that bound in the beach, over which there was only a winding rugged footpath towards Lerici, and none on the other side; the tideless sea leaving no sands nor shingle, formed a picture such as one sees in Salvator Rosa's landscapes only. Sometimes the sunshine vanished when the sirocco raged – the 'ponente' the wind was called on that shore. The gales and squalls that hailed our first arrival surrounded the bay with foam; the howling wind swept round our exposed house, and the sea roared unremittingly, so that we almost fancied ourselves on board ship. At other times sunshine and calm invested sea and sky, and the rich tints of Italian heaven bathed the scene in bright and ever-varying tints.

The natives were wilder than the place. Our near neighbours of San Terenzo were more like savages than any people I ever before lived among. Many a night they passed on the beach, singing, or rather howling; the women dancing about among the waves that broke at their feet, the men leaning against the rocks and joining in their loud wild chorus. We could get no provisions nearer than Sarzana, at a distance of three miles and a half off, with the torrent of the Magra between; and even there the supply was very deficient. Had we been wrecked on an island of the South Seas, we could scarcely have felt ourselves farther from civilisation and comfort; but, where the sun shines, the latter becomes an unnecessary luxury, and we had enough society among ourselves. Yet I confess housekeeping became rather a toilsome task, especially as I was suffering in my health, and could not exert myself actively.

At first the fatal boat had not arrived, and was expected with great impatience. On Monday, 12th May, it came. Williams records the long-wished-for fact in his journal: 'Cloudy and threatening weather. M. Maglian called; and after dinner, and while walking with him on the terrace, we discovered a strange sail coming round the point of Porto Venere, which proved at length to be Shelley's boat . . . She does indeed excite my surprise and admiration. Shelley and I walked to Lerici, and made a stretch off the land to try her: and I find she fetches whatever she looks at. In short, we have now a perfect plaything for the summer.' – It was thus that short-sighted mortals welcomed Death, he having disguised his grim form in a pleasing mask! The time of the friends was now spent on the sea; the weather became fine, and our whole party often passed the evenings on the water when the wind promised pleasant sailing. Shelley and Williams made longer excursions; they sailed several times to Massa . . .

The heats set in in the middle of June; the days became excessively hot. But the sea-breeze cooled the air at noon, and extreme heat always put Shelley in spirits. A long drought had preceded the heat; and prayers for rain were being put up in the churches, and processions of relics for the same effect took place in every town. At this time we received letters announcing the arrival of Leigh Hunt at Genoa. Shelley was very eager to see him. I was confined to my room by severe illness, and could not move; it was agreed that Shelley and Williams should go to Leghorn in the boat. Strange that no fear of danger crossed our minds! Living on the sea-shore, the ocean became as a plaything: as a child may sport with a lighted stick, till a spark inflames a forest, and spreads destruction over all, so did we fearlessly and blindly tamper with danger, and make a game of the terrors of the ocean. Our Italian neighbours, even, trusted themselves as far as Massa in the skiff; and the running down the line of coast to Leghorn gave no more notion of peril than a fair-weather inland navigation would have done to those who had never seen the sea. Once, some months before, Trelawny had raised a warning voice as to the difference of our calm bay and the open sea beyond; but Shelley and his friend, with their one sailor-boy, thought themselves a match for the storms of the Mediterranean, in a boat which they looked upon as equal to all it was put to do.

On the 1st of July they left us. If ever shadow of future ill darkened the present hour, such was over my mind when they went. During the whole of our stay at Lerici, an intense presentiment of coming evil brooded over my mind, and covered this beautiful place and genial summer with the shadow of coming misery. I had vainly struggled with these emotions – they seemed accounted for by my illness; but at this hour of separation they recurred with renewed violence. I did not antici-pate danger for them, but a vague expectation of evil shook me to agony, and I could scarcely bring myself to let them go. The day was calm and clear; and, a fine breeze rising at twelve, they weighed for Leghorn. They made the run of about fifty miles in seven hours and a half. The 'Bolivar' was in port; and, the regulations of the Health-office not permitting them to go on shore after sunset, they borrowed cushions from the larger vessel, and slept on board their boat.

They spent a week at Pisa and Leghorn. The want of rain was severely felt in the country. The weather continued sultry and fine. I have heard that Shelley all this time was in brilliant spirits. Not long before, talking of presentiment, he had said the only one that he ever found infallible was the certain advent of some evil fortune when he felt peculiarly joyous. Yet, if ever fate whispered of coming disaster, such inaudible but not unfelt prognostics hovered around us. The beauty of the place seemed unearthly in its excess: the distance we were at from all signs of civilization, the sea at our feet, its murmurs or its roaring for ever in our ears, – all these things led the mind to brood over strange thoughts, and, lifting it from everyday life, caused it to be familiar with the unreal. A sort of spell surrounded us; and each day, as the voyagers did not return, we grew restless and disquieted, and yet, strange to say, we were not fearful of the most apparent danger.

The spell snapped; it was all over; an interval of agonizing doubt – of days passed in miserable journeys to gain tidings, of hopes that took firmer root even as they were more baseless – was changed to the certainty of the death that eclipsed all happiness for the survivors for evermore . . . A year before [Shelley] had poured into verse all such ideas about death as give it a glory of its own. He had, as it now seems, almost anticipated his own destiny . . . his skiff wrapped from sight by the thunder-storm, as it was last seen upon the purple sea, and then, as the cloud of the tempest passed away, no sign remained of where it had been . . .

Captain Roberts watched the vessel with his glass from the top of the lighthouse of Leghorn, on its homeward track. They were off Via Reggio, at some distance from shore, when a storm was driven over the sea. It enveloped them and several larger vessels in darkness. When the cloud passed onwards, Roberts looked again, and saw every other vessel sailing on the ocean except their little schooner, which had vanished. From that time he could scarcely doubt the fatal truth; yet we fancied that they might have been driven towards Elba or Corsica, and so be saved.

The observation made as to the spot where the boat disappeared caused it to be found, through the exertions of Trelawny for that effect. It had gone down in ten fathom water; it had not capsized, and, except such things as had floated from her, everything was found on board exactly as it had been placed when they sailed. The boat itself was uninjured. Roberts possessed himself of her, and decked her; but she proved not seaworthy, and her shattered planks now lie rotting on the shore of one of the Ionian islands, on which she was wrecked. Who but will regard as a prophecy the last stanza of [Shelley's] 'Adonais'?

'The breath whose might I have invoked in song
Descends on me; my spirit's bark is driven,
Far from the shore, far from the trembling throng
Whose sails were never to the tempest given;
The massy earth and sphered skies are riven!
I am borne darkly, fearfully, afar;
Whilst burning through the inmost veil of Heaven,
The soul of Adonais, like a star,
Beacons from the abode where the Eternal are.'

Putney, May 1, 1839.

~

MATTHEW WEBB BECAME THE FIRST person to swim the English Channel without aids on 25 August 1875, an achievement which stood unique until 1911. For a time after this, Webb – who became a merchant mariner at the age of twelve, and had been awarded bravery medals for trying to save a fellow sailor who fell overboard during an Atlantic gale – was a celebrity. But recognition for his near twenty-two hours of Channel swimming did not bring him lasting prosperity. Instead, Webb eked out a living giving lectures and performing displays, which consisted of him swimming up and down a tank at a stately pace for – in one case sixty – hours, but over time the crowds shrank and he struggled to support his wife and young family.

In 1883, Webb sought to renew his fame by swimming across the whirlpool rapids below Niagara Falls, an impossible feat. His body, undoubtedly crushed by the staggering weight of the water, was never found, but still his wife Madeline for many years hoped he would return. John Betjeman, poet laureate in the 1970s, wrote this songlike tribute to Webb, who was born in Dawley in the English county of Shropshire, borrowing its title from A. E. Housman's collection.

'Paying a call at Dawley Bank while swimming along to Heaven.'
'A Shropshire Lad' by John Betjeman[82]

The gas was on in the Institute,
The flare was up in the gym,
A man was running a mineral line,
A lass was singing a hymn,
When Captain Webb the Dawley man,
Captain Webb from Dawley,
Came swimming along the old canal
That carried the bricks to Lawley.
Swimming along –
Swimming along –
Swimming along from Severn,
And paying a call at Dawley Bank while swimming along to Heaven.

The sun shone low on the railway line
And over the bricks and stacks
And in at the upstairs windows
Of the Dawley houses' backs

When we saw the ghost of Captain Webb,
Webb in a water sheeting,
Come dripping along in a bathing dress
To the Saturday evening meeting.
Dripping along –
Dripping along –
To the Congregational Hall;
Dripping and still he rose over the sill and faded away in a wall.

There wasn't a man in Oakengates
That hadn't got hold of the tale,
And over the valley in Ironbridge,
And round by Coalbrookdale,
How Captain Webb the Dawley man,
Captain Webb from Dawley,
Rose rigid and dead from the old canal
That carries the bricks to Lawley.
Rigid and dead –
Rigid and dead –
To the Saturday congregation,
Paying a call at Dawley Bank on the way to his destination.

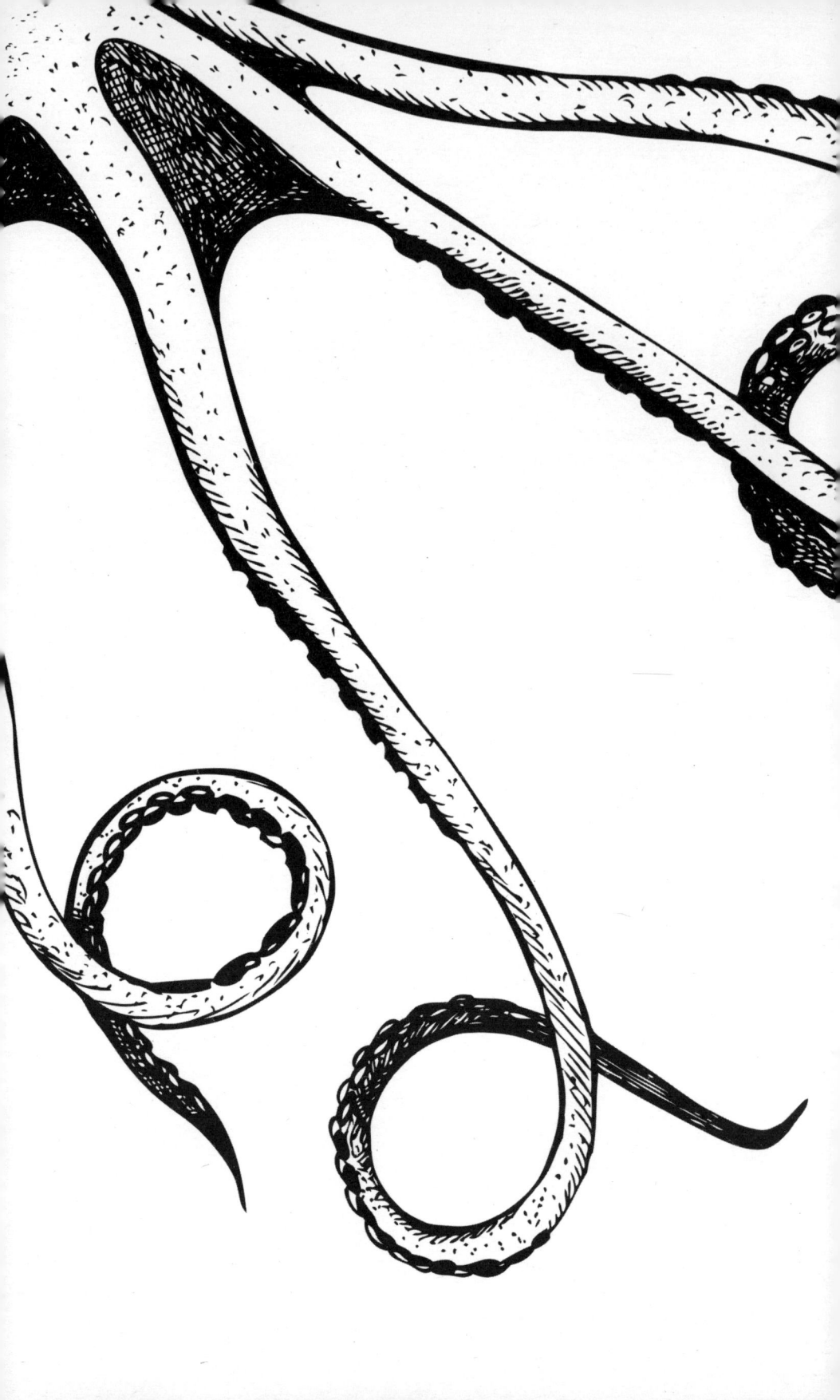

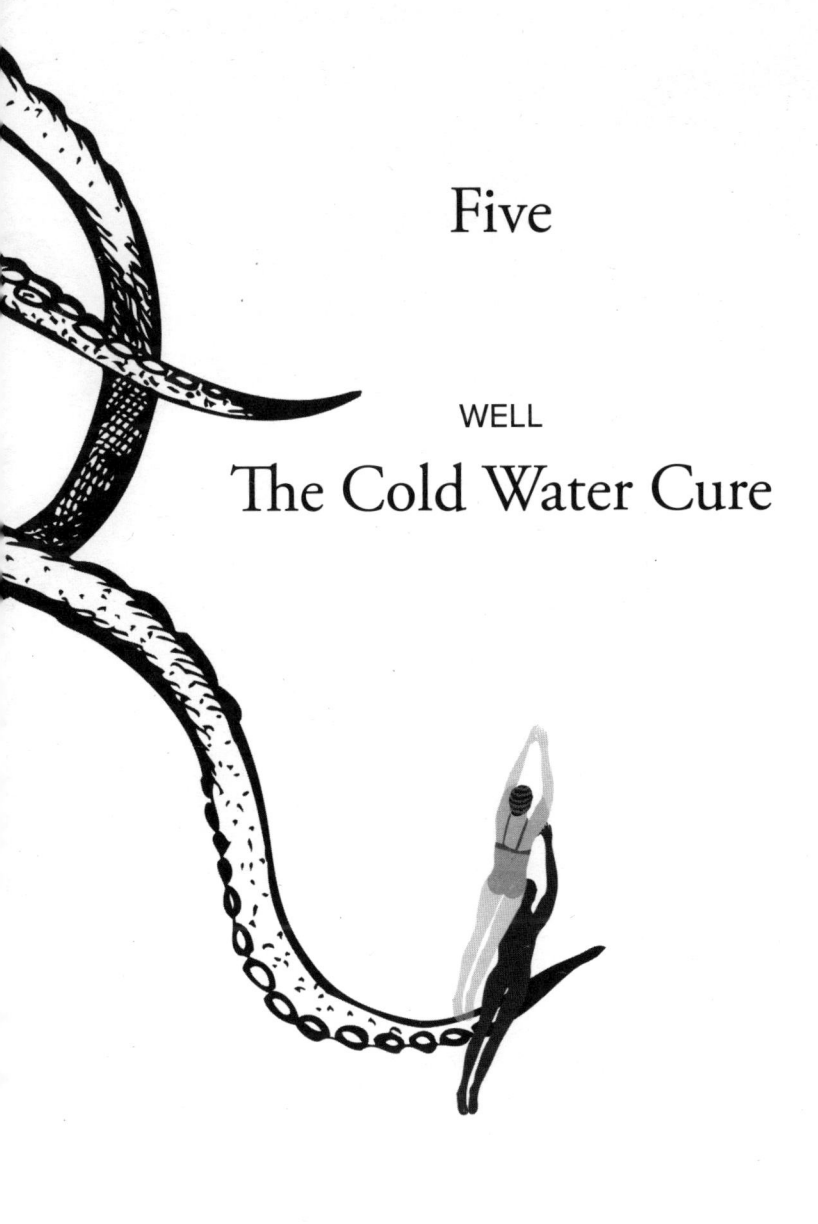

Five

WELL

The Cold Water Cure

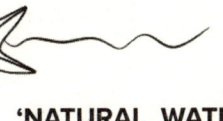

'NATURAL WATER,' THE SWIMMER and environmentalist Roger Deakin wrote in his turn-of-the-century memoir of swimming across Britain 'has always held the magical power to cure.'

I'm not one of those people who went to the sea looking for a cure, but over the years I've noticed how swimming has borne me through difficult times. It was, for instance, bobbing around on Lough Mask in Ireland, staring up at an infinity of grey, that I found solace after the death of my brother. It felt as if he was somewhere out there in that sky, or in the water that held me so lightly. Not long after, when the menopause hit me sideways and off guard, the thrill of immersion in cold water, of being body-slammed by the waves, picked me up.

So, when I started wild swimming it was not because I had heard of its benefits, but, as I began working on my first swim book, *Taking The Plunge*, with Anna Deacon, I did start to hear of them, in a torrent of compelling testimonies from people who had arrived at the water and discovered some remarkable health boosts.

Around the same time, I noticed that there were books, some old, but mostly new, telling the story of the transformational magic of a swim in the wild. Authors like Roger Deakin, originator of the term 'wild swimming', or Ruth Fitzmaurice, who found the sea and a tribe to support her as she struggled with caring for her husband Simon, who had motor neurone disease.

I found myself going for the odd literary dip, or clocking the odd passage on swimming in whatever book I was reading, or even re-calling, on my swims, a scene from a book read long ago.

This reminded me that, of course, the 'wild' bit of swimming is nothing new. We humans have been swimming, in all parts of the world, for millennia. We only have to look back through all of our literatures – and our art and music, too – to find the tales, the stories of love, amusement, exhilaration, physicality and daring.

But we talk about it differently now. We speak of its physiological and emotional benefits. We rave about the science of 'cold water immersion'; how cold water shock exercises the sympathetic nervous system, or how the dive reflex sparks the vagus nerve; we discuss how research is increasingly showing that cold water dipping may help treat certain conditions, from depression through to diabetes; we are excited to discover how this activity is so good for us that, perhaps, it should even be made a 'public health measure'. But it's also worth remembering when we come to talking about whether swimming outdoors delivers health benefits, there are two factors that have been essential to the narrative for millennia – and these are the cold and nature. They are part of a story that begins long in the past and takes us through to now.

In Britain, after decades of cheap flights, package holidays and heated swimming pools, it feels as if a generation has come back to their local sea, lakes and rivers, and indeed the cold. That feeling of something new-found is there in an extraordinary wave of writing about swimming – and not just about swimming itself, but about the way in which it has changed our lives, and can alter who we are.

But that feeling is not entirely new. As some of the passages in this section show, we have been here before.

CHAPTER I

Recovery

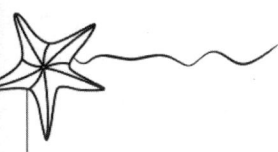

ONE OF THE RECURRENT STORIES around how swimming changes us is recovery – whether from life's harshest blows, its sorrows and losses, illness or addiction. In so much writing, the water is where we recover, or where we recover something of ourselves. It restores us to ourselves and others.

Greystones in County Wicklow, Ireland is a reminder for me of this. I've swum five or six times at the snug, sea-swept cove with the embracing community of swimmers who take a daily sunrise dip in its swells and, though I have never met the author Ruth Fitzmaurice, I've often thought of her book, *I Found My Tribe*, when I am there. This gut-wrenching, captivating memoir tells of caring for her husband Simon (1973–2017) through his devastating decline with motor neurone disease, and how she found solace and solidarity in the Irish Sea. It's a reminder of how water can bring release and intense togetherness.

'My cove is my tribe and the tribe is mine.'
I Found My Tribe by Ruth Fitzmaurice[83]

My husband is a wonder to me but he is hard to find. I search for him in our home. He breathes through a pipe in his throat. He feels everything but cannot move a muscle. I lie on his chest counting mechanical breaths. I hold his hand but he doesn't hold back. His darting eyes are the only windows left. I won't stop searching. My soul demands it and so does his. Simon has motor neurone disease, but that's not the dilemma, at least not today. Be brave.

In the midst of this, she begins to go down to the sea . . .

There was a blood moon last night and the sea is agitated. My soul is agitated. The full moon gets a red glow during a lunar eclipse, says Marian, so watch out. Blood moons belong to moongazers, dreamers and to Marian. For them, the night sky is a realm of intense feeling and romance. I'd never heard of such things, so I lean in closer. We are up to eighty per cent water, Marian says, and that is why the moon and the tides affect us. That is why I jump in the sea, I say. I am trying to find a home, make a home, *be* a home for my five children. Sometimes I succeed and sometimes I fail.

The story she tells is a search for, and finding of, belonging.

My friend's calm cousin cuts through the bullshit. 'Find your tribe,' she says. Finding your people is more important than what kind of house you live in. Decide whether you've found your tribe and go from there. I believe her.

My cove is my tribe and the cove is mine. My babies stand with soggy shoes on the shore, skidding on wet stones and cheer as their Momma plunges to her salvation. Yes, this is my cove and the sea is my salvation. It shocks my body back to life, as rain darts on the sea surface on a misty, romantic day.

She also describes the complicated range of feelings she experiences while in the water:

> But on another day I stood at the edge of the sea and wept. My feet were submerged on the bottom step and I wiggled my red toenails and sobbed. My sea-swimming friend was there to hug me. The sea was choppier but my soul was calmer and refreshed and content when I climbed back up the steps. We may be eighty per cent water, Marian, I think, but my emotions are as mysterious to me as the swell of the sea. All I know is that I could never leave this place. The cove is my tribe and the sea saves me.

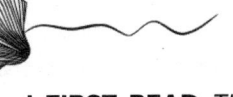

I FIRST READ *The Outrun* by Amy Liptrot on holiday in Orkney a couple of years ago. My husband, Rob, was dealing with the after-effects of a serious bout of Covid, specifically a more or less constant sensation of seasickness, which we later discovered to be vestibular neuritis. We'd rented a cottage on one of the islands in the archipelago, which was without internet or Wi-Fi. It was June, and the weather was cool and overcast. Rob spent a lot of time lying in ditches, watching birds and cloudscapes. Our wee but and ben was on a half-moon bay of white sand and I swam there each morning, feeling a bit like Robinson Crusoe arriving on a deserted shore when I emerged from the bracing water.

Before we took the ferry, from the Orkney mainland to the isle of Stronsay, I borrowed a pile of books from Kirkwall Library, including this, Amy Liptrot's first. The isle was a perfect place to read *The Outrun*. The title refers to what Orcadians call the field at the far edge of the farm or croft, often close to the sea cliff. In it, Liptrot tells of her return to her childhood home in search of healing after becoming an alcoholic in London in her twenties. That part of the book includes a description of breaking into a swimming pool at night with her boyfriend.

Liptrot drinks so much on the boat back to Orkney that she has to be helped to disembark. When she dries out, she takes a job monitoring corncrake numbers and describes obsessively driving around in the night, winding down her car windows to listen for this small and secretive bird's characteristic call. Immersing herself in cold water is also part of her new life. Later, Liptrot joins a wild swimming group called the Polar Bears, which takes her another step towards recovery.

'I want to shock myself awake.'

The Outrun by Amy Liptrot[84]

I prepare by eating porridge and listening to aggressive rap. We make a strange group: undressing car side into swimming costumes, woolly hats and goosebumps. Going sea swimming with a group provides the motivation that is lacking when you're alone. Everyone has different techniques for getting into the water, some running enthusiastically, others repeatedly edging up to genital level before backing out . . .

We swim in windscreen-wipers-on highest setting rain when we rush to get into the water where it's dryer. We're lifted by the bow waves of passing boats. The water is always different: dark and velvety, sometimes perfectly clear, flat and glassy. We swim when sunshine dapples the surface and illuminates bubbles underwater.

On 1 May, in celebration of May Day or Beltane, we meet at dawn, five-fourteen a.m. at the most easterly beach on the Orkney Mainland, where we can see the sun rise over the ocean horizon. The sea is black and thick when we walk in, but as the sun rises, it lights our laughing, yelping faces and catches the rippling waves. We swim on the minute of the summer solstice at the north coast of the Mainland, just after midnight at 12:09 a.m. when it is still light in the grimlins. The next morning I smell of bonfire smoke and taste of sea salt. Following the points of the compass and the turning points of the year, we go to the west coast for sunset on Lammas, an ancient celebration of the first harvest.

It's a misty night with no sunset and it's spooky in the geo, where we slip on seaweed and my fellow swimmers are half shrouded in the fog. I was on Papay when the group swam after dark on the winter solstice, wearing head torches, guided back to the shore by a light on the beach. It feels ritualistic, this celebration of solstices and equinoxes, following compass points, moon and tide charts and sunrise calendars.

I didn't realise until I was back in Orkney and more aware of these things, but the day after my last drink – my first day sober – was the spring equinox, 20 March. Since then, each solstice and equinox has marked another quarter-year of sobriety. I enjoy this: it links my small choices and individual behaviour into the patterns of the solar system. The swims are a way to celebrate.

It is always gaspingly cold. The sea temperature gets gradually higher all summer, to an average of a cold thirteen degrees in September; then, when the air temperature becomes cooler than the water, it goes down to an 'extremely cold' four or so degrees in February. The first time felt like it was burning my skin but each Saturday it gets slightly easier – your body acclimatises – although I am the wimpiest member of the club, back onshore drying myself while the others are still breast-stroking around the pier. It's a convivial group, heads up, chatting while we swim.

I want to shock myself awake: after central heating and screens, to feel cold, with skin submerged in wild waters, is attractively physical. I want to blast away the frustrations of being stuck on this island and no longer have the outlet of getting drunk. The chilly immersion is addictive, verging on unpleasant at the time, but I find myself craving it, agreeing to go again, planning my next swim, eyeing up lochs, bays or reservoirs. I want to swim in bomb craters.

During each of the first few swims there is a point when my body panics. I picture drowning and, knowing the depth beneath me, my heart rate increases. I need to reach the shore as quickly as possible. When I do pull myself out up the slipway, climbing the ladder onto the pier, or washing up with the waves onto the beach, I feel saved: reborn and very alive.

People claim all sorts of health benefits from wild swimming – better circulation, improved immunity – with the Outdoor Swimming Society pledging to 'embrace the rejuvenating effects of cold water' but I mainly do it for the 'cold-water high', the exhilaration and endorphins resulting from even a short dip.

Afterwards, I go about my Saturday – first stop the supermarket – with a crazy smile and bright red salty skin. Other Polar Bears report an increase of energy to start the weekend but one member told me she just enjoys that other people think she's mad. It's an unconventional hobby and a weekly adventure.

THE STORIES PEOPLE TELL ABOUT how swimming helps us, even saves us, have been central to the books I have created with photographer Anna Deacon. That which some perceive as madness is not only joyful, but supports our sanity. Among them is this tale told by Kenny Neilson who went from being obliterated by his alcoholic benders to setting up a cold water therapy community, the Polar Bear Club.

'I was a lost boy.'
The Ripple Effect by Anna Deacon and Vicky Allan[85]

Kenny Neilson on the Polar Bear Club

I woke up in hospital after a serious suicide attempt. In that time, I'd built a massive business in the gas industry. I had ten guys working for me. I was getting flown backwards and forwards down to London. But I drank my nights away. I never spoke to my weans, never spoke to my partner. I was isolating in my room every night, getting up in the morning going to work, coming home and drinking till I passed out. That came to a head on Halloween 2021.

I knew twelve-step back to front. But knowledge is irrelevant. Action is everything – and I wasn't putting it into action. So, having a head full of that and a belly full of swally, I was in total meltdown. That Halloween, I couldn't take it anymore and I couldn't stop drinking. I was lost. I had all this knowledge, but I couldn't stop. I had a litre of Morgan's Spice that I'd got as a present when I started my business. I put it all in two big tumblers, and I thought if I drink these two in a oner, I'll never wake up again. So, I gubbed them and woke up in hospital the next morning, thinking, What has happened?

I was a lost boy. When the psychologist assessed me, they said, 'You know there's nothing we can do for you. There's nothing anyone can do for you. You're as well running back to your meetings.' And that's what I did. I went back to my meetings.

I'd already tried the water. About nine months prior, my sponsor from twelve-step took me up into the Campsies in the middle of winter when it was snowing and he put me in the water.

Then, around December, after I had come out of the hospital in October, my big mate said to me, want to try the cold water again? He took me up to the Campsies. I went in and this time I was sober and searching for something. The thing is, with the programme, you're searching for a god of your own understanding, a power you can talk to and hold inside yourself. But being a scheme boy, I was like what is a god? I couldn't understand it. How can I find a god? I don't know nothing about religion.

But when he put me in the water, something came over me. My head went blank. I couldn't think and it was beautiful. I sat in the water and embraced the cold. It was December and freezing, but I was in the zone with it. And I made the decision that day to shut the business down. I paid the guys off and never did another day's work for about four or five months.

In that waterfall, I was searching for a god. I was praying and I was trying my hardest. I was in the water screaming, 'Please, God, don't make me drink today!' I was broken. I was at a moment of desperation. In that moment in the water when I felt the cold seeping into me, it came to me like that, You're going to be alright. You're going to be alright. Then I started laughing. I was howling to myself. I thought to myself, See, if someone was walking down there and saw me, they'd be saying, 'Who is this big bam?' They'd be going, 'God save me!'

I came out of the water that day and I felt like I'd been plugged into nature. I'd been plugged into my surroundings, plugged into the cold water, plugged into the deep breathing. And the next morning I woke up and I prayed. I prayed to Mother Nature.

I began the Polar Bear Club after I started sharing what I was experiencing on social media. I started turning my camera on when I went into the water and saying, 'Look what's happening everybody.' I felt the craving for alcohol was gone. I've cleared my head and I'm no longer craving it because I'm no longer drinking it.

~

IN HER 2023 MEMOIR, FREYA BROMLEY recounts a year spent swimming in every tidal pool in Britain, using wild swimming as a tool for processing her grief at losing her brother Tom, who died of cancer at the age of nineteen.

'Everything passes by, I thought.'
The Tidal Year by Freya Bromley[86]

Grantchester Meadows: 52.1810° N, 0.0932° E
I woke up that Thursday in a single bed in Madingley Hall. My insides ached. There was a lump in my throat like a knot in wood and a tension in my temples hinted I needed to cry, but I knew if I started, I wouldn't be able to stop. Some days grief was like that.

I took two steps to the window and stared at the hedgerows. I tried to think of the birds that might be outside: blue tit, sparrow, greenfinch, Tom. I took three steps to the bathroom and washed my face. The tap made a juddering sound when it started and the water smelled ancient.

For four days I'd been staring at the page, writing poems and working. I'd lift my pen and the letters to form his name would appear. TOM. As a little boy, Tom struggled to master writing his name and wrote it backwards. We called him Motty. I used to draw dots on his page so he could join them together.

It was all so painful; I couldn't write anything past his name. I wanted to try in case it was the answer, so I got back into bed, put my laptop on my chest and opened Word. I hovered over the T button, which was waiting right beneath my index finger. The cursor blinked at me. I hit 'Exit and Discard Changes', although there were none to 'Save'.

I thought about Miri; I missed her. I wondered what she'd say right now. Probably, go have a swim. Recently it'd felt like there was lots she'd told me I couldn't do, but maybe I could try this one. I typed 'Swim Cambridge' into the search bar. Jesus Green Lido wasn't far, but it didn't open till 7 a.m. and the booking app looked like it was made on Microsoft Publisher 1997. I booked an Uber to Grantchester Meadows, which involved reassuring the driver that just here is fine please, despite his reservations about why a girl wanted to be dropped off by the river so early.

I walked to a bend in the River Cam and found a wooden ladder. It was simple. It was quiet. It was perfect. There was an orange fire in the sky, dawn had arrived. I undressed quickly. A ruffling in the marshes signalled I'd disturbed a brown hare enjoying its morning by the water. The flamed sky was mirrored on the still pool of water and the meadow blazed with wildflowers. Knapweed, ox-eye daisies, field scabious and meadow buttercups still in bloom. I slipped into the brown water and my heart beat fast, a radiating thud. thud. I heard it in my ears and remembered that I was alive, which often felt like an accidental detail. Blood was being pumped around my body at four miles an hour. I would keep going.

A cloud of white floated onto the river. I stayed still, treading water, wondering if I should fear the swan. Her wings were folded by her sides, but I knew if she lifted them her strength could overpower me. She made the slightest movement of her beak, almost curious, which I took to mean she was content sharing the river.

I inhaled deeply, then placed my head under the water and screamed. Bubbles escaped my mouth like I'd boiled the water with my anger. Jem was right, it helped the rage. I sensed the beat of wings as a trio of birds fled the reeds. My entire face felt frozen, jaw stuck.

Standing by a cluster of yellow fieldcap mushrooms, I peeled my sodden underwear from my body. I was ill-equipped for emerging from the swim and only had a white towel from Madingley Hall that was streaked with brown mud once I'd dried myself. I took a moment to just be, then, as the mist cleared, I walked away from the river.

CHAPTER II

The Doctor's Line

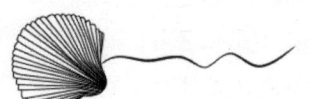

HISTORY IS FULL OF THOSE who knew the water's magic – writers and rulers, alike – and it only takes a little digging to find them. Emperor Charlemagne, the Holy Roman Emperor, who ruled much of Western Europe in the eighth century, was so convinced of the healing powers of water that he moved his capital to what we now call Aachen at the juncture of where Germany meets Belgium and the Netherlands. There he built a sumptuous palace, and the town is still a spa today – one of the best-known in Europe.

The medieval scholar Einhard wrote a biography of his patron, who died in 814 AD, at seventy-two, a good old age for medieval times. Many will sympathise with the Emperor's attitude to medical advice.

'A hundred or more persons sometimes bathed with him.'
The Life of Charlemagne by Einhard[87]

His health was excellent, except during the four years preceding his death, when he was subject to frequent fevers; at the last he even limped a little with one foot. Even in those years, he consulted rather his own inclinations than the advice of physicians, who were almost hateful to him, because they wanted him to give up roasts, to which he was accustomed, and to eat boiled meat instead. In accordance with the national custom, he took frequent exercise on horseback and in the chase, accomplishments in which scarcely any people in the world can equal the Franks.

He enjoyed the exhalations from natural warm springs, and often practised swimming, in which he was such an adept that none could surpass him; and hence it was that he built his palace at Aix-la-Chapelle, and lived there constantly during his latter years until his death. He used not only to invite his sons to his bath, but his nobles and friends, and now and then a troop of his retinue or body guard, so that a hundred or more persons sometimes bathed with him.

THE MEDICINAL PRACTICE OF IMMERSION in cold water for health and enjoyment goes way back. The saunas, complete with cold plunge, that we associate with the Nordic countries and which are now part of a hot shoreline trend in the UK, are thought to have originated about 2,000 BCE. But the earliest surviving writing about this practice is from the Greek physician Hippocrates, who recommended immersion in either warm or cold water for various conditions in about 400 BCE. The Romans advised following a warm bath with a cold one, to maintain health and vigour. The Chinese physician Hua To, in the second century, recommended the pouring of a hundred buckets of cold water over the patient as a cure for fever. Hua would not have been impressed by the modern craze known as the ice bucket challenge.

Swimming was common in the ancient world. But there was a period when most Europeans didn't swim. Superstitions grew in the north of the continent in the early modern period, perhaps influenced by the regional Little Ice Age, which began in the thirteenth century. People began to believe that water had metaphysical properties and that entering its depths could disturb spirits. And, of course, the 'sink or float' test of 'swimming' was used to determine whether a woman was a witch, along with the infamous 'ducking stool' which was used to drench – and silence – the 'common scold'.

By the sixteenth century, many European authorities, including the University of Cambridge, were issuing edicts that made swimming illegal.

But Cambridge don Everard Digby went against the grain and produced a book of swimming tips in 1587. A rebellious character, Digby was deprived of his fellowship the same year, partly because of his heterodox views and partly on account of his habit of blowing a horn and shouting in college. Some of Digby's swimming advice seems dubious – perhaps best not tried at your local river, even if it is the Cam.

'To pare his toes in the water.'

A Short introduction for to learne to Swimme by Everard Digby[88]

To pare his toes in the water.

Swimming upon his back, let him draw up his left foot, and lay it over his right knee, still keeping his body very straight and then having a knife ready in his right hand, he may easily keep up his leg until he hath pared one of his toes . . .

GRADUALLY, PHYSICIANS ACROSS Europe rediscovered the benefits of cold bathing for health. Among them was John Floyer who, in his 1706 treatise, describes how the practice was already deeply rooted in history.

'I do esteem Cold Bathing a very ancient as well as useful Practice.'

Psychrolousia. Or, *The History of Cold Bathing* by John Floyer[89]

Bathing in Rivers, and the Sea, was most Ancient for Exercise, Pleasure, and curing Diseases. A place for swimming in Cold Water was provided for in the Roman Baths, and was more Ancient than they. The manner of the Romans was to conclude their Hot Bathing with the Cold Water; which shews the good Opinion they had of Cold Immersion.

And to assert the Usefulness and Safety of the Cold Baths, I could instance in Augustus and Horace, who used them by the Advice of Musa. Pliny and Seneca testify of the Use of them; and Lampridiusy that the Emperor Severus practised Cold Bathing for the Gout. And that Cold Baths were anciently used in England, may be proved, because all the Northern Nations used that Method for fortifying themselves against their Cold Air.

The Art of Cold Bathing was certainly first Invented by the Common People, who used it for the Preservation of their Health, and fortifying themselves against Cold, as other Animals do. The Priests farther improved this by applying it to Divine Immersion, thereby to purify the Spirits, and to make them more Calm and Vigorous in Devotion.

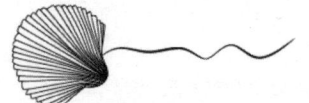

FLOYER WAS AN EARLY VOICE in a trend that would sweep Europe over the course of the eighteenth century and would develop into the modern hydrotherapy movement. But some doctors thought the therapy's benefits exaggerated, even dangerous.

That was the view of an eminent Scottish doctor who questioned the wisdom of a colleague in an earlier era who had suggested the poet Robert Burns should go sea-bathing.

There are still people who are sceptical of the benefits of wild swimming, some of whom see it as a great way of exposing yourself to the pathogens of the UK's creaky sewage system, or an equally great way of catching your death of cold. Certain newspaper columnists like to rail against the perceived idiocy of wild swimming. Jeremy Clarkson described it as practically suicidal, arguing that nature is far from clean and that open water is full of decaying matter and parasites. This view would probably find a sympathetic hearing from Sir James Crichton-Browne.

Crichton-Browne, an eminent psychiatrist and one of Charles Darwin's collaborators, scrutinised this regimen and period of the poet's life, in *Burns From a New Point of View*, based on a series of articles in the *Glasgow Herald* and first published as a book in 1925 (when its author was eighty-five). He quotes at length from letters which show Burns was troubled in mind as well as body, tormented by money worries and anxiety for his family in those last days at the spa. Burns returned from Brow-Well just two days before his death on 21 July 1796.

'The medical people order me, as I value my existence, to fly to sea-bathing.'

Burns From a New Point of View by James Crichton-Browne[90]

Ten miles south-east of Dumfries on the Solway shore stands the meanest, shabbiest little spa in all the world. It consists of three white-washed cottages, a tank the size of a dining table, and lined with red sandstone, into which through an iron pipe the mineral water trickles, an esplanade a score of yards long of coarse tufted grass, and the pump-room, a dilapidated wooden shed, the walls and benches of which are graven over and over again with the initials of those who have sought healing at the well.

The country immediately around is flat and uninteresting. Inland there are a few stunted plantations of gnarled oaks and shaggy Scotch firs, which by their bent backs bear witness to the rough usage of the western winds, while in front there is a broad fat hillocky expanse, studded with bent grass and furze, and ending in the sea-beach, consisting of a mixture of sand and clay, known locally as sleetch. This uninviting substance extends for several miles into the Solway Firth. with so slight a declination that the tide at low water recedes entirely out of sight, and leaves to the eye a barren and cheerless waste . . . But, whatever its physical features may be, the Brow-Well must be regarded as a sacred precinct by all Scotsmen, for it was the scene of the last act of a memorable and deeply Scottish tragedy. It was the Gethsemane of Robert Burns. It was here that 'exceeding sorrowful even unto death' he spent the last fortnight of his glorious but troubled life.

Why was Burns sent to the Brow-Well? Looking back from the medical point of view on the meagre reports of his state of health which have come down to us, it seems clear that his regimen there was the worst possible under the circumstances and hastened his end.

Dr Maxwell no doubt acted for the best, but he took . . . an entirely erroneous view of Burns's case, and, thinking, as Burns says he did, that melancholy and low spirits were half his disease, he suggested change of scene, the drinking of water which was regarded as tonic . . . the restorative influence of country quarters and. incredible as it may seem, considering his condition, of sea-bathing and of exercise on horseback.

Dr Maxwell long afterwards represented to Dr Currie that Burns was impatient of medical restraint, and determined himself to try the effects of sea-bathing; but Burns expressly says, 'The medical people order me, as I value my existence, to fly to sea-bathing and country quarters.'

So this broken-down man, who had seldom left his house for months and had spent most of his time in bed, who could scarcely stand upon his legs and bore on his countenance the pale cast of death, was sent to bathe in the open sea of the Solway, where bathing is, at its best, only possible for two weeks in the month, owing to the state of the tides, and even then after much wading to obtain any depth of water. He was also to bestride and jolt about on a Rosinante.

Brow-on-Solway, 4th July 1796.

My Dear Sir,—I received your songs; but my health is so precarious, nay, dangerously situated, that, as a last effort, I am here at sea-bathing quarters. Besides an inveterate rheumatism, my appetite is quite gone, and I am so emaciated as to be scarce able to support myself on my own legs. Alas! Is this a time for me to woo the muses? However, I am still anxiously willing to serve your work, and if possible shall try. I would not like to see another employed—unless you could lay your hand upon a poet whose productions would be equal to the rest. Farewell, and God bless you.

To his father-in-law, Burns wrote:

My wife is hourly expecting to be put to bed. Good God! what a situation for her to be in, poor girl, without a friend. I return from sea-bathing quarters today, and my medical friends would almost persuade me that I am better, but I think and feel that my strength is so gone that the disorder will prove fatal to me.

Crichton-Browne concludes:

Callous must be the man who could read these letters without a rising in his throat. The pity, the shame of it, to think of this sublime, glorious genius, the kindest-hearted poet that ever lived, stricken with mortal disease in his prime, and still, say what they may, in full possession of choice gifts, to think of him at that supreme hour harassed by sordid cares and haunted by ghastly apprehensions!

CHAPTER III

Taking the Waters

BATHING WAS EMBRACED BY MEN and women of letters – as it was by the characters they created in their novels. The spa or watering place became a feature of life – at least for the middle and upper classes. But one of the earliest literary spa descriptions is this amusing episode by the Scottish poet Tobias Smollett that evokes the Yorkshire town of Scarborough, in his epistolary novel *The Expedition of Humphry Clinker*, first published in 1771. An elderly landowner, Matthew Bramble, and his family are on a trip around Scotland, along with a manservant, Humphry Clinker, that they have picked up along the way.

These days dry robes are all the rage – as well as provoking a certain amount of rage among those who, in the title of one social media page, dub their wearers 'dry robe wankers' or write the garments off as middle-class status symbols. But back then it was these changing huts on wheels.

Scarborough was home to the very first bathing machine, designed to deliver the swimmer to and from the sea in supposedly perfect modesty and dignity. Dignity, however, is hardly what is brought to mind in this passage, told in a letter from the point of view of Bramble's nephew, Jeremy Melford.

'The bather, ascending into this apartment by wooden steps, shuts himself in, and begins to undress.'
The Expedition of Humphry Clinker by Tobias Smollett[91]

From Harrigate, we came hither, by the way of York, and here we shall tarry some days, as my uncle and Tabitha are both resolved to make use of the waters. Scarborough, though a paltry town, is romantic from its situation along a cliff that overhangs the sea . . . Betwixt the well and the harbour, the bathing machines are ranged along the beach, with all their proper utensils and attendants.

You have never seen one of these machines — Image to yourself a small, snug, wooden chamber, fixed upon a wheel-carriage, having a door at each end, and on each side a little window above, a bench below — The bather, ascending into this apartment by wooden steps, shuts himself in, and begins to undress, while the attendant yokes a horse to the end next the sea, and draws the carriage forwards, till the surface of the water is on a level with the floor of the dressing-room, then he moves and fixes the horse to the other end — The person within being stripped, opens the door to the sea-ward, where he finds the guide ready, and plunges headlong into the water — After having bathed, he re-ascends into the apartment, by the steps which had been shifted for that purpose, and puts on his clothes at his leisure, while the carriage is drawn back again upon the dry land; so that he has nothing further to do, but to open the door, and come down as he went up — Should he be so weak or ill as to require a servant to put off and on his clothes, there is room enough in the apartment for half a dozen people.

The guides who attend the ladies in the water, are of their own sex, and they and the female bathers have a dress of flannel for the sea; nay, they are provided with other conveniences for the support of decorum.

A certain number of the machines are fitted with tilts, that project from the sea-ward ends of them, so as to screen the bathers from the view of all persons whatsoever — The beach is admirably adapted for this practice, the descent being gently gradual, and the sand soft as velvet; but then the machines can be used only at a certain time of the tide, which varies every day; so that sometimes the bathers are obliged to rise very early in the morning . . .

Your affectionate friend and servant,

J. Melford. Scarborough, July 1

In the next letter Matthew Bramble, the ailing, somewhat hypochondriac patriarch in pursuit of a spa cure, attempts a plunge in the sea.

I went down to the bathing-place, attended by my servant Clinker, who waited on the beach as usual — The wind blowing from the north, and the weather being hazy, the water proved so chill, that when I rose from my first plunge, I could not help sobbing and bawling out, from the effects of the cold. Clinker, who heard me cry, and saw me indistinctly a good way without the guide, buffetting the waves, took it for granted I was drowning, and rushing into the sea, clothes and all, overturned the guide in his hurry to save his master. I had swam out a few strokes, when hearing a noise, I turned about and saw Clinker, already up to his neck, advancing towards me, with all the wildness of terror in his aspect — Afraid he would get out of his depth, I made haste to meet him, when, all of a sudden, he seized me by one ear, dragged me bellowing with pain upon the dry beach, to the astonishment of all the people, men, and women, and children there assembled.

I was so exasperated by the pain of my ear, and the disgrace of being exposed in such an attitude, that, in the first transport I struck him down; then, running back into the sea, took shelter in the machine where my clothes had been deposited. I soon recollected myself so far as to do justice to the poor fellow, who, in great simplicity of heart, had acted from motives of fidelity and affection — Opening the door of the machine, which was immediately drawn on shore, I saw him standing by the wheel, dropping like a water-work, and trembling from head to foot; partly from cold, and partly from the dread of having offended his master — I made my acknowledgments for the blow he had received, assured him I was not angry, and insisted upon his going home immediately, to shift his clothes; a command which he could hardly find in his heart to execute, so well disposed was he to furnish the mob with further entertainment at my expence. Clinker's intention was laudable without all doubt, but, nevertheless, I am a sufferer by his simplicity — I have had a burning heat, and a strange buzzing noise in that ear, ever since it was so roughly treated; and I cannot walk the street without being pointed at; as the monster that was hauled naked a-shore upon the beach.

~

SEVENTY-FIVE YEARS OR SO LATER, Queen Victoria used bathing machines like the ones Smollett described – though without any mishap involving her being dragged naked ashore.

'I thought it delightful till I put my head under water, when I thought I should be stifled.'

Queen Victoria's journal, Friday 30 July 1847[92]

A very fine morning, & the day became again very hot . . . drove down to the beach with my maids & went into the bathing machines, where I undressed & bathed in the sea, (for the 1rst time in my life) a very nice bathing woman attending me. I thought it delightful till I put my head under water, when I thought I should be stifled. After dressing again, drove back.

~

TWO OF JANE AUSTEN'S COMPLETED novels are set in spa towns, *Northanger Abbey* in Bath and *Persuasion* in Lyme Regis. These watering places were then at the height of their popularity with all kinds of claims being made for the health benefits of sea air, mineral water and sea bathing. Austen's last, unfinished book, *Sanditon*, also uses the water cure as a backdrop. Here Mr Parker, a passionate believer in the promise of the spa claims that sea air and sea bathing are, together, 'infallible'.

There is always comedy in a thing that becomes a fashion and, in the nineteenth century, Austen was not alone in taking a swipe. One popular souvenir publication, *Twelve Subjects of the Water Cure*, featured engravings of the 'horrors' of a patient undergoing hydrotherapy, including one in which he is sprayed by a hose with the caption: 'This is how we are treated, as if we are garden shrubs.'

Another, *Pleasures of the Water Cure* by the illustrator and satirist Thomas Onwhyn, sees a terrified patient approached with a 'wet sheet' and bucket, declare, 'But I am sure I shall get my death of cold.'

Even the novelist Charles Dickens, inspired by his visits to Malvern Wells in pursuit of rehabilitation for his wife Catherine's supposed 'nervous illness' (perhaps post-partum depression), wrote a one-act play, *Mr. Nightingale's Diary*. The farce is centred on a hypochondriac in search of a cold water cure, whose complaint, says one character, is 'nothing'.

'He'll never get over it, sir,' replies another. 'Of all the invalids that come down here, the invalids that have nothing the matter with them are the hopeless cases.'

'If the sea breeze failed, the sea-bath was the certain corrective.'

Sanditon by Jane Austen[93]

He wanted to secure the promise of a visit, to get as many of the family as his own house would contain, to follow him to Sanditon as soon as possible; and, healthy as they all undeniably were, foresaw that every one of them would be benefited by the sea. He held it indeed as certain that no person could be really well, no person (however upheld for the present by fortuitous aids of exercise and spirits in a semblance of health) could be really in a state of secure and permanent health without spending at least six weeks by the sea every year.

The sea air and sea bathing together were nearly infallible, one or the other of them being a match for every disorder of the stomach, the lungs or the blood. They were anti-spasmodic, anti-pulmonary, anti-septic, anti-billious and anti-rheumatic. Nobody could catch cold by the sea; nobody wanted appetite by the sea; nobody wanted spirits; nobody wanted strength. Sea air was healing, softening, relaxing fortifying and bracing seemingly just as was wanted sometimes one, sometimes the other. If the sea breeze failed, the sea-bath was the certain corrective; and where bathing disagreed, the sea air alone was evidently designed by nature for the cure . . .

'Before we accept your hospitality sir, and in order to do away with any unfavourable impression which the sort of wild-goose chase you find me in may have given rise to, allow me to tell you who we are. My name is Parker, Mr. Parker of Sanditon; this lady, my wife, Mrs. Parker. We are on our road home from London. My name perhaps, though I am by no means the first of my family holding landed property in the parish of Sanditon, may be unknown at this distance from the coast. But Sanditon itself—everybody has heard of Sanditon. The favourite for a young and rising bathing-place, certainly the favourite spot of all that are to be found along the coast of Sussex—the most favoured by nature, and promising to be the most chosen by man.'

'Yes, I have heard of Sanditon,' replied Mr. Heywood. 'Every five years, one hears of some new place or other starting up by the sea and growing the fashion. How they can half of them be filled is the wonder! Where people can be found with money and time to go to them! Bad things for a country—sure to raise the price of provisions and make the poor good for nothing—as I dare say you find, sir.'

'Not at all, sir, not at all,' cried Mr. Parker eagerly. 'Quite the contrary, I assure you. A common idea, but a mistaken one. It may apply to your large, overgrown places like Brighton or Worthing or Eastbourne but *not* to a small village like Sanditon, precluded by its size from experiencing any of the evils of civilization, while the growth of the place, the buildings, the nursery grounds, the demand for everything and the sure resort of the very best company whose regular, steady, private families of thorough gentility and character who are a blessing everywhere, excited the industry of the poor and diffuse comfort and improvement among them of every sort. No sir, I assure you, Sanditon is not a place—'

'I do not mean to take exception to any place in particular,' answered Mr. Heywood. 'I only think our coast is too full of them altogether. But had we not better try to get you—'

'Our coast too full!' repeated Mr. Parker. 'On that point perhaps we may not totally disagree. At least there are enough. Our coast is abundant enough. It demands no more. Everybody's taste and everybody's finances may be suited. And those good people who are trying to add to the number are, in my opinion, excessively absurd and must soon find themselves the dupes of their own fallacious calculations. Such a place as Sanditon, sir, I may say was wanted, was called for. Nature had marked it out, had spoken in most intelligible characters. The finest, purest sea breeze on the coast—acknowledged to be so—excellent bathing— fine hard sand—deep water ten yards from the shore—no mud—no weeds—no slimy rocks. Never was there a place more palpably designed by nature for the resort of the invalid—the very spot which thousands seemed in need of!'

Jane Austen loved sea bathing – but it did not prevent her from succumbing to a mystery illness at the age of forty-one in 1817. Medics disagree about what caused the much-loved writer's early death – everything from Addison's disease to breast cancer has been proposed. They also disagree about whether the liveliness and wit of her prose indicates that she was in good health prior to her last illness. Can someone battling ill health be funny? Of course, funnier than the well perhaps. And if Jane was something of a sceptic about the power of the cold water cure, maybe it was because she knew from experience it could not vanquish her own fatigue.

When they were apart, Jane wrote often to her beloved elder sister Cassandra, and sometimes mentioned sea bathing – she may have mentioned it in other correspondence, but we don't know. Cassandra destroyed most of Jane's letters in an attempt to preserve her privacy, a story told in a novel by Gill Hornby and a BBC TV series *Miss Austen*.

**'I continue quite well: in proof of which
I have bathed again this morning.'**
A letter from Jane Austen to her sister Cassandra, from Lyme,
September 1804[94]

You found my letter at Andover, I hope, yesterday, and have now for many hours been satisfied that your kind anxiety on my behalf was as much thrown away as kind anxiety usually is. I continue quite well: in proof of which I have bathed again this morning. It was absolutely necessary that I should have the little fever and indisposition which I had: it has been all the fashion this week in Lyme.

A few days later, she continued:

Friday Evening. The bathing was so delightful this morning and Molly so pressing with me to enjoy myself that I believe I staid in rather too long, as since the middle of the day I have felt unreasonably tired. I shall be more careful another time, and shall not bathe tomorrow as I had before intended.

~

CHARLOTTE BRONTË WAS DOING IT too. In 1852, she travelled to Filey, a fishing village with a long beach near Scarborough, to visit the grave of her sister Anne.

'I have bathed once – it seemed to do me good.'
The Life of Charlotte Brontë by Elizabeth Gaskell[95]

Charlotte wrote to her father:

I have not bathed yet as I am told it is too cold and too early in the season. The sea is very grand. Yesterday was a somewhat unusually high tide – and I stood about an hour on the cliffs yesterday afternoon – watching the tumbling in of great tawny turbid waves – that make the whole shore white and filled the air with a sound hollower and deeper than thunder . . . When the tide is out – the sands are wide – long and smooth and very pleasant to walk on.

And to her lifelong friend Ellen Nussey:

Cliffe House, Filey, June 6th, 1852.

Dear E—,

I am at Filey utterly alone. Do not be angry, the step is right. I considered it, and resolved on it with due deliberation. Change of air was necessary; there were reasons why I should not go to the south, and why I should come here. On Friday I went to Scarborough, visited the churchyard and stone. It must be refaced and relettered; there are five errors. I gave the necessary directions. That duty, then, is done; long has it lain heavy on my mind; and that was a pilgrimage I felt I could only make alone.

I am in our old lodgings at Mrs. Smith's; not, however, in the same rooms, but in less expensive apartments. They seemed glad to see me, remembered you and me very well, and, seemingly, with great good will. The daughter who used to wait on us is just married. Filey seems to me much altered; more lodging-houses – some of them very handsome – have been built; the sea has all its old grandeur. I walk on the sands a good deal, and try not to feel desolate and melancholy. How sorely my heart longs for you, I need not say.

I have bathed once; it seemed to do me good. I may, perhaps, stay here a fortnight. There are as yet scarcely any visitors. A Lady Wenlock is staying at the large house of which you used so vigilantly to observe the inmates. One day I set out with intent to trudge to Filey Bridge, but was frightened back by two cows. I mean to try again some morning. I left papa well. I have been a good deal troubled with headache, and with some pain in the side since I came here, but I feel that this has been owing to the cold wind, for very cold has it been till lately; at present I feel better. Shall I send the papers to you as usual? Write again directly, and tell me this, and anything and everything else that comes into your mind. – Believe me, yours faithfully,

C. Brontë

CHAPTER IV

Literally Wild

WRITERS COULD ALSO BE INFLUENCERS, changing the culture of their time, and many embraced open water swimming for mental and physical health. Henry David Thoreau was what we might call a lifestyle guru. In the mid-nineteenth century, he based himself in a hut he built in the New England countryside. He lived in a self-sufficient way and later produced a best-selling book of essays, *Walden*, which combines nature writing with homilies about how people – mainly scientific, manly people – should live. One of the delights of his life there was starting each day with a dip in the pond.

'I got up early and bathed at the pond.'
Walden by Henry David Thoreau[96]

Every morning was a cheerful invitation to make my life of equal simplicity, and I may say innocence, with Nature herself. I have been as sincere a worshipper of Aurora as the Greeks. I got up early and bathed in the pond; that was a religious exercise, and one of the best things which I did. They say that characters were engraven on the bathing tub of King Tchingthang to this effect: 'Renew thyself completely each day; do it again, and again, and forever again.' I can understand that.

Morning brings back the heroic ages . . . The morning, which is the most memorable season of the day, is the awakening hour. Then there is least somnolence in us; and for an hour, at least, some part of us awakes which slumbers all the rest of the day and night.

Little is to be expected of that day, if it can be called a day, to which we are not awakened by our Genius, but by the mechanical nudgings of some servitor; are not awakened by our own newly acquired force and aspirations from within, accompanied by the undulations of celestial music, instead of factory bells, and a fragrance filling the air – to a higher life than we fell asleep from.'

Thoreau would generally take a second bathe after working:

After hoeing, or perhaps reading and writing, in the forenoon, I usually bathed again in the pond, swimming across one of its coves for a stint, and washed the dust of labor from my person, or smoothed out the last wrinkle which study had made, and for the afternoon was absolutely free.

~~~

GEORGE SAND WAS THE PEN NAME of Amantine Lucile Aurore Dupin de Francueil, one of the most celebrated European novelists of the nineteenth century. Sand, who wore male attire in public, was more famous than the renowned Romantic author of *Les Misérables*, Victor Hugo, during her lifetime. She wrote regularly to Gustave Flaubert, who often referred to her as a member of 'the third sex'. Both loved swimming and here Sand describes her daily swim.

'Regaining my strength in this cold and shady stream.'
The George Sand–Gustave Flaubert Letters, translated by Aimee L. McKenzie[97]

George Sand To Gustave Flaubert, at Caoisset
Nohant, 10 September, 1867

Dear old fellow,

I am worried at not having news of you since that illness of which you spoke. Yes, we shall go to see the rollers and the beaches next month if you like, if your heart prompts you. The novel goes on apace; but I shall besprinkle it with local colour afterwards.

While waiting, I am still here, stuck up to my chin in the river every day, and regaining my strength entirely in this cold and shady stream which I adore, and where I have passed so many hours of my life reviving myself after too long sessions in company with my ink-well.

The era ends with this Kafka-esque diary entry from Franz Kafka himself on the outbreak of the Great War. Kafka loved swimming, and when a doctor recommended that he should take a break because of his heart problems, he wrote to his fiancée Felice Bauer: 'Not swim? That's impossible!'

It's a reminder that, for some, the simple act of swimming has been taking place as part of the backdrop of the most monumental events of life and of history. In his diary, Kafka wrote, 'Sunday, August 2, 1914: Germany has declared war on Russia. Swimming in the afternoon.'

CHAPTER V

Rediscovery

OVER THE TWENTIETH CENTURY, SWIMMING became something people, particularly in chillier countries, did in heated – and chlorinated – pools in controlled conditions with lifeguards, lanes, opening hours and a whole world of etiquette. It was still valued for exercise and relaxation but it became a tamer, more predictable and decorous affair than it had been – and also more of a competitive sport.

For naturalist and author Roger Deakin, swimming in open water was essentially subversive, a break with the norm of his day. He loved immersing himself in nature in this way and found it could shift his mood from dark to light in a moment. Deakin's bewitching travel book, *Waterlog*, in which he swims across Britain via its rivers and waterways, did much to inspire the culture of open water swimming in the UK. The book begins by recognising the power of water.

'There is a feeling of absolute freedom and wildness.'
Waterlog by Roger Deakin[98]

Natural water has always held the magical power to cure. Somehow or other, it transmits its own self-regenerating powers to the swimmer. I can dive in with a long face and what feels like a terminal case of depression, and come out a whistling idiot. There is a feeling of absolute freedom and wildness that comes with the sheer liberation of nakedness as well as weightlessness in natural water, and it leads to a deep bond with the bathing-place. Most of us live in a world where more and more places and things are signposted, labelled, and officially 'interpreted'.

There is something about all this that is turning the reality of things into virtual reality. It is the reason why walking, cycling and swimming will always be subversive activities. They allow us to regain a sense of what is old and wild in these islands, by getting off the beaten track and breaking free of the official version of things. A swimming journey would give me access to that part of our world which, like darkness, mist, woods or high mountains, still retains most mystery. It would afford me a different perspective on the rest of land-locked humanity.

IN THE MIDDLE OF THE sprawling city of London are three freshwater ponds with changing rooms and lifeguards where people can swim outdoors. The first time I ever visited the Mixed Pond on Hampstead Heath, I swam, one warm summer day, with a new friend, and we lay on the grass afterwards and fell asleep listening to the buzz of insects. I felt like I had gone tumbling down the rabbit hole.

Whenever I have been since, it has felt like diving through a portal, in the midst of the city, to another space, both strange and wonderful. For many, of course, the Hampstead ponds are their routine swim spot, described lovingly and intimately for instance in the collected, multi-authored essays of *At the Pond: Swimming at the Hampstead Ladies' Pond*, and also in a journal published in 2015 by poet and non-fiction writer Al Alvarez.

'That's one of the fascinations of these ponds; they, too, are bits of wild nature in the middle of town.'
Pondlife: A Swimmer's Journal by Al Alvarez[99]

Monday 16 December. 40°F
I love these dark mornings. The midwinter solstice is approaching, cars still have their headlights on at 9.30 in the morning, the Heath is deserted, the water is as black as Grendel's lake and very cold. When you dive in, everything contracts to the centre to keep the core warm, then flows outwards again when you get out. Hence the lobster flush, or, if you prefer, the healthy glow. I suppose this determination to survive adversity was something I picked when I was operated on as a baby and the need to test myself constantly followed from it. Whatever the cause, it's now a habit of mind that makes me feel fully alive, second only to making love to Anne. The obligatory cold baths at Oundle every morning gave me the taste for cold water and I went on taking them the following year in that freezing little cottage that I shared with the school butler when I was teaching at Maidwell Hall. Rock climbing – feeding the rat – was a natural progression.

Sunday 28 September. 60°F
A slow and beautiful autumn, coming on by minute degrees. Today the water is a little fresher than yesterday and the breeze a little cooler, though not really enough to notice. There have been a few showers and it gets dark earlier, but the mornings feel lazy and warm enough out of the wind; the only chill comes up through your feet from the concrete. And the seagulls are back. They seem suddenly to be everywhere, eyeing you coldly as you swim, skimming low over your head, circling, calling. Just before I dived in yesterday the heron zoomed low over the water

on its great clattering wings. Seeing him is always a sudden pleasure – I suppose because it seems so strange to meet such a shy, wild creature here in the middle of London. But, then, that's one of the fascinations of these ponds; they, too, are bits of wild nature in the middle of town and, when winter comes, wild, cold and relatively untamed. What would I do without them?

~~~~~

A BODY OF WATER CHANGES through the seasons. In *Turning*, nature writer and environmental historian Jessica J. Lee captures the thrill so many of us feel swimming in open water as the temperature starts to drop.

'Even in winter, the lake is alive beneath the ice.'
Turning: Lessons from Swimming Berlin's Lakes by Jessica J. Lee[100]

A swimmer can sense the turning of the lake. There's a moment in the season when the water changes. It isn't something you can see, it's something you can feel. In spring, the winter ice melts, and the warm and cold of the lake intermingle, flowing together. In summer, as the lake grows warm, a green froth of algae caps the surface of the water, and when it cools again in autumn, the green disappears. The air thins. The leaves flash red and gold. And the water 'turns'.

You come to know the consistent cool of spring and the stagnant warmth at the top of a summer lake. When the water clears in the autumn, you can feel it: the lake feels cleaner on your arms, less like velvet and more like cut glass. And then winter comes, sharper than ever. Swimming year-round means greeting the lake's changes.

There is an English expression for the lake's changes: the 'breaking of the meres'. It describes the point in late summer when shallow lakes – meres – turn a turbid blue-green, algae breaking atop the surface like yeast froths on beer. The Germans also have a word for the green of summer: umkippen. It describes the point when the water has turned to slick green, fizzling with iridescent algae.

But the breaking of the meres and umkippen capture only that single moment of algal rupture, the death of the lake from too much algae and too little oxygen. We tend to notice the obvious thing – the emerging sheen of an algal bloom – and reduce a word's meaning to that tiny moment, that fleck of green on the surface.

The lake's turning – 'lake stratification' and 'overturn' – runs deeper, taking in an entire year's worth of changes in the water. Turning is perpetual. It points to the wider transformations in the water, as layers below billow and rearrange themselves beneath the surface. Even in winter, the lake is alive beneath the ice.

I long for the ice. The sharp cut of freezing water on my feet. The immeasurable black of the lake at its coldest. Swimming then means cold, and pain, and elation.

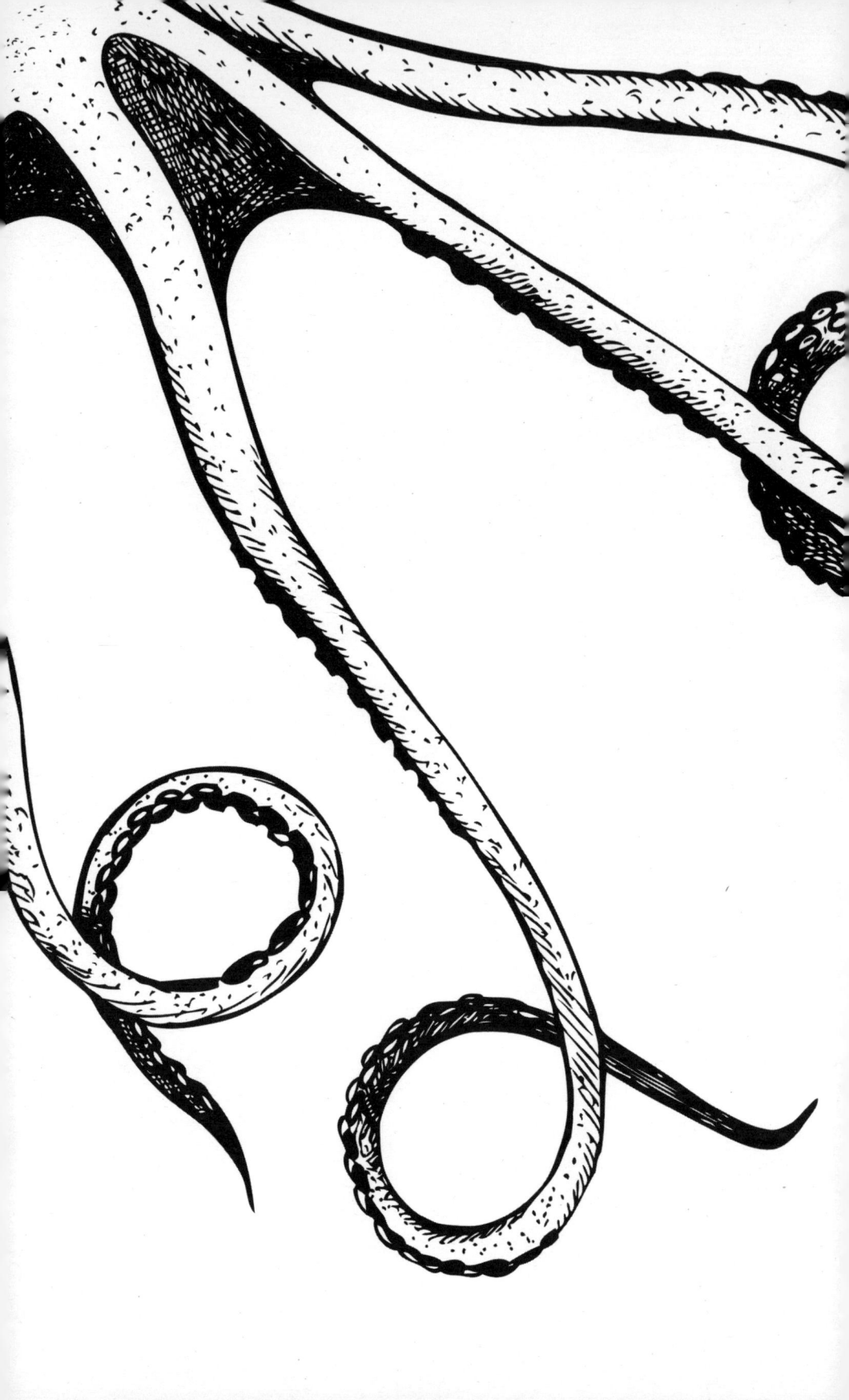

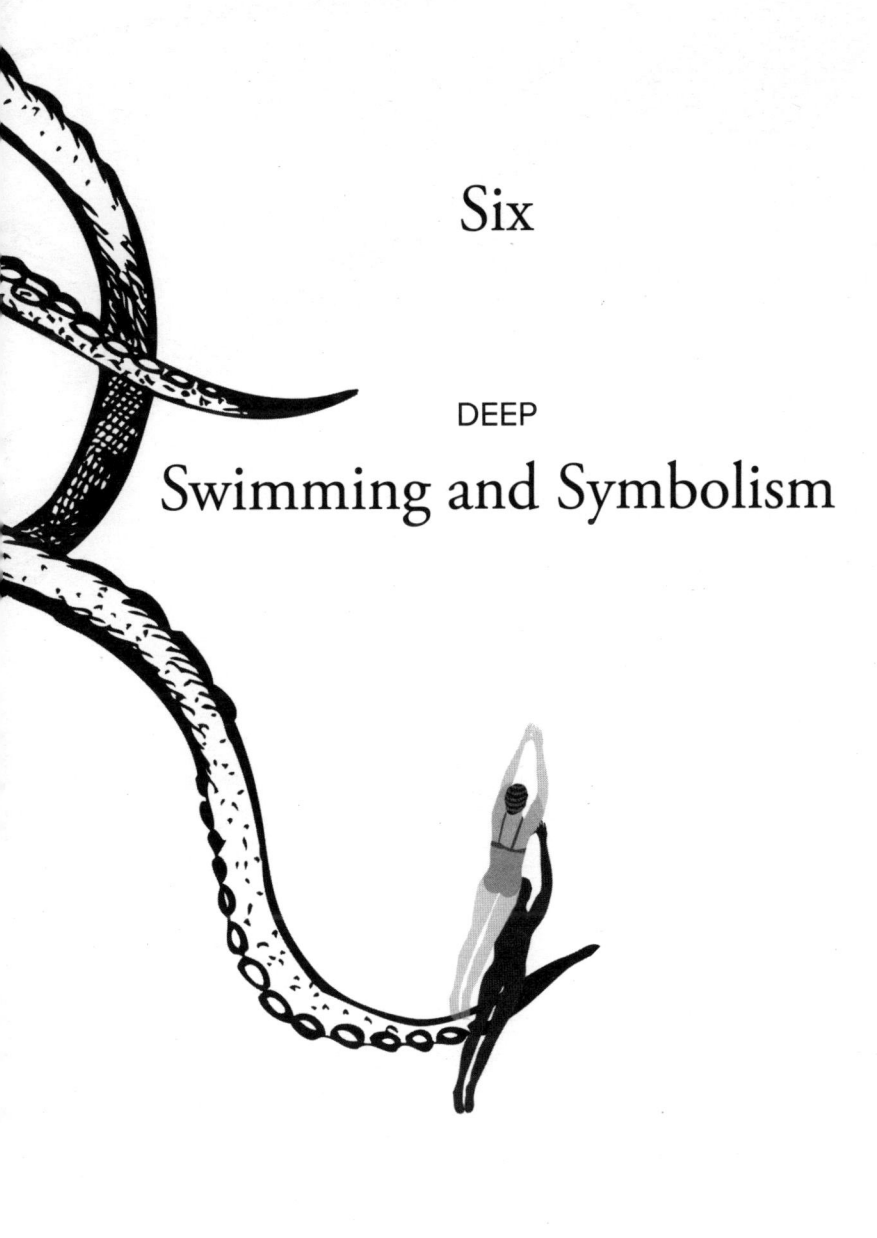

Six

DEEP

Swimming and Symbolism

SYMBOLISM PERMEATES OUR RELATIONSHIP WITH the water. The psychoanalyst Carl Jung described the sea as the 'favourite symbol for the unconscious, the mother of all that lives'. The sea or the river can represent life's flow; the journey in dark water can be a plunge down into the underworld. In the wild ocean of our language, shoals of metaphors swim.

Once you start noticing them, you see them everywhere.

I'll always remember how, when I was first panicking over whether I could write my first swimming book to a very tight deadline, psycho-therapist and swimmer, Ange Cameron said to me, 'You know how to ride a wave. You've ridden them before. You can ride this one.'

What I've also learned from speaking with swimmers is that we carry what we learn from the sea, or from other waters, including the chlorinated blue rectangles of the pool, into our lives. Just as cross-country runners, say, carry the knowledge of the hills and moors with them. My photographer-collaborator on many swimming books, Anna Deacon and I would often talk about how similar the challenge of public speaking was to immersion into cold water. We would get the fear, want to back out, but then plunge in, do what we needed to do – practised, but almost instinctive too – and ultimately emerge from those icy waters abuzz with life. If we could face a choppy, chill sea, we told ourselves, we could do this.

There is a fascination in the metaphors we use around swimming and the way that the physical experience can help us tackle and process difficult feelings, especially grief. When I spoke with Ange about the solace I had found in the water around my sorrow for my brother, she said: 'The waves are like grief. They come and go in their strength and intensity. There's something so predictably unpredictable about the sea and that's not too dissimilar to grief.'

Ange also spoke of how sometimes she took people, struggling with grief, depression or anxiety, into the sea. 'If people have lost their way, they've reached a place where they're not able to find meaning in their life, I find to go into the elements of the sea can have a profound effect and bring us back to life.'

CHAPTER I

Océanique

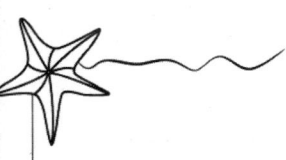

SOME OF THE MOST REMARKABLE stories I came across in researching my wild swimming books were from people who felt they had experienced an almost baptismal transformation in the water. One of these was featured in *Swimming Wild Ireland!*

'At that point, I was terrified of water.'
Swimming Wild Ireland! by Anna Deacon and Vicky Allan[101]

Ciara McCormack's story

The day it happened, I went down for my walk on the beach along Dunany coast. I can't remember how I even ended up there, but I went into the water fully clothed in the depths of a cold winter morning. I came out of the water that day a very different person. It changed my whole perspective on life forever. I had to completely reprogramme myself.

A few weeks beforehand, I had been thinking about it being my time to go. I thought, I didn't belong here. I was not worthy. That was my thought process. I went into that sea thinking that I had no purpose in this world.

All this happened to me in November 2019 just before the Covid pandemic. My husband at the time, now ex, had an affair which was the catalyst for a massive shift to happen in my life. I had been in a very abusive, co-dependent marriage for 17 years. When you are in a marriage with a narcissist you don't see it until you step out of the picture and get clarity on everything. And that is what I did, because abuse becomes normalised, and you start to doubt yourself. I felt I was going crazy. The threats I endured, one being: 'If you walk out of here, I'll make your life hell and I'll take the kids.' And that was exactly what he did.

As a mother and a wife, my whole world collapsed. I suffered from serious PTSD. I didn't know what it was at the time or what was going on in my life. I couldn't sleep, I couldn't eat, and I couldn't function anymore and, to top it off, Covid had just begun. I've had some traumatic experiences in my life. I was raped in my twenties in a restaurant in London. I was abused by a family member when I was a very young child. But this chapter of my life was the worst. Having one's children taken away is hard for any mother but knowing what was ahead for my children was harder for me as I always protected them and knew that the cycle of abuse with my ex was going to begin again, this was my breaking point.

At a very young age, I was terrified of water. My father had taken me into the small harbour in the village where I grew up. He was a strong swimmer and a diver and I almost drowned in the water that day, so my fear of water was off the charts. I couldn't go in without panicking. I had such a fear of water even on holiday. I would panic at the mere thought of going into the sea. I would only go in up to my knees and my panic attacks would start. But there I was on that day in November in the coldest of water, fully clothed and looking at myself, so calm and being able to breathe.

At that point in my life, I was at rock bottom. I remember being on Dunany Cliff that morning standing there, thinking, 'Which rock to jump off?'

I don't remember thinking about suicide when I walked into the sea. I felt almost like I was guided into the water. I thought, 'What has just happened?' I couldn't explain it, I wasn't cold, I was able to breathe and my heart felt so much love and warmth. I now realise that it was a new chapter for me, a new beginning, the water had completely cleansed me. It was all so aligned, like the universe was saying I belong here and I have work to do for others.

I went into the water again the next day and every day after that, and I guess now it's my fuel for life. Sometimes our fears become our strengths. I carried so much fear from my childhood which completely set me back my whole life, the moment I would put my feet in the water, my breath would accelerate and I would just start panicking.

Our whole life is a stage. Sometimes it can take an overwhelming breakdown to have an undeniable breakthrough in life. We are the directors and we have the power to change our script. I feel all the things that have happened throughout my life are preparing me for every moment that is yet to come. All the versions of you that you didn't love, brought you to the versions of you that you love now, so be grateful for the different people you have been.

IN SOMETIMES LIGHT-HEARTED RECOGNITION OF the water's life-enhancing power, swimmers often quip that their dip is a baptism, or they might call their regular weekly swim a 'Sunday Service' (a moniker shared by other sports, admittedly), or even claim that, as one swimmer told me, 'John the Baptist was the world's first wild swimmer.' Scenes inspired by these feelings of religiosity and transformation often feature in novels.

An unconventional baptism by the edge of a river is a pivotal scene in Marilynne Robinson's Pulitzer Prize-winning 'Gilead' trilogy, a love story between an older, widowed preacher and a homeless woman. In the first book, John Ames, supposedly writing for the child they have together, whom he knows he will not live to see grow up, discusses the meaning of baptism – and of water.

'Shimmer and splash.'
Gilead by Marilynne Robinson[102]

Ludwig Feuerbach says a wonderful thing about baptism. I have it marked. He says, 'Water is the purest, clearest of liquids; in virtue of this, its natural character, it is the image of the spotless nature of the Divine Spirit. In short, water has a significance in itself, as water; it is on account of its natural quality that it is consecrated and selected as the vehicle of the Holy Spirit. So far there lies at the foundation of Baptism a beautiful, profound natural significance.' Feuerbach is a famous atheist, but he is about as good on the joyful aspects of religion as anybody, and he loves the world. Of course, he thinks religion could just stand out of the way and let joy exist pure and undisguised. That is his one error, and it is significant. But he is marvelous on the subject of joy, and also on its religious expressions

That mention of Feuerbach and joy reminded me of something I saw early one morning a few years ago, as I was walking up to the church. There was a young couple strolling along half a block ahead of me. The sun had come up brilliantly after a heavy rain, and the trees were glistening and very wet. On some impulse, plain exuberance, I suppose, the fellow jumped up and caught hold of a branch, and a storm of luminous water came pouring down on the two of them, and they laughed and took off running, the girl sweeping water off her hair and her dress as if she were a little bit disgusted, but she wasn't. It was a beautiful thing to see, like something from a myth. I don't know why I thought of that now, except perhaps because it is easy to believe in such moments that water was made primarily for blessing, and only secondarily for growing vegetables or doing the wash. I wish I had paid more attention to it. My list of regrets may seem unusual, but who can know that they are, really. This is an interesting planet. It deserves all the attention you can give it.

In writing this, I notice the care it costs me not to use certain words more than I ought to. I am thinking about the word 'just'. I almost wish I could have written that the sun just shone and the tree just glistened, and the water just poured out of it and the girl just laughed – when it's used that way it does indicate a stress on the word that follows it, and also a particular pitch of the voice. People talk that way when they want to call attention to a thing existing in excess of itself, so to speak, a sort of purity or lavishness, at any rate something ordinary in kind but exceptional in degree. So it seems to me at the moment. There is something real signified by that word 'just' that proper language won't acknowledge. It's a little like the German ge-. I regret that I must deprive myself of it. It takes half the point out of telling the story . . .

You and Tobias are hopping around in the sprinkler. The sprinkler is a magnificent invention because it exposes raindrops to sunshine. That does occur in nature, but it is rare. When I was in seminary I used to go sometimes to watch the Baptists down at the river. It was something to see the preacher lifting the one who was being baptized up out of the water and the water pouring off the garments and the hair. It did look like a birth or a resurrection. For us the water just heightens the touch of the pastor's hand on the sweet bones of the head, sort of like making an electrical connection. I've always loved to baptize people, though I have sometimes wished there were more shimmer and splash involved in the way we go about it. Well, but you two are dancing around in your iridescent little downpour, whooping and stomping as sane people ought to do when they encounter a thing so miraculous as water.

~

SIGMUND FREUD – THE PSYCHOANALYST MOST strongly associated with the concept of the unconscious mind – argued that dreams of swimming are often connected to birth. Here, he analyses a patient's dream of swimming.

'She hurls herself into the dark water at a place where the pale moon is reflected in the water.'
The Interpretation of Dreams by Sigmund Freud[103]

Here is a pretty water-dream of a female patient, which was turned to extraordinary account in the course of treatment. At her summer resort at the . . . Lake, she hurls herself into the dark water at a place where the pale moon is reflected in the water.

Dreams of this sort are parturition dreams; their interpretation is accomplished by reversing the fact reported in the manifest dream content; thus, instead of 'throwing one's self into the water,' read 'coming out of the water,' that is, 'being born.' The place from which one is born is recognised if one thinks of the bad sense of the French 'la lune.' The pale moon thus becomes the white 'bottom' (Popo), which the child soon recognises as the place from which it came. Now what can be the meaning of the patient's wishing to be born at her summer resort? I asked the dreamer this, and she answered without hesitation: 'Hasn't the treatment made me as though I were born again?' Thus the dream becomes an invitation to continue the cure at this summer resort, that is, to visit her there; perhaps it also contains a very bashful allusion to the wish to become a mother herself . . .

ONE OF THE FIRST MEMOIRS I read from the new wave of books about wild swimming, Victoria Whitworth's captivating and illuminating *Swimming with Seals*, touches in a key chapter on some of Freud's thinking. I was struck by her descriptions of how, in the water, she felt part of something bigger and would feel herself 'dissolving'.

'I tread water and hold my breath, but not as long as the seal does.'
Swimming with Seals by Victoria Whitworth[104]

Oh, hello.

This encounter always triggers the same response: a little twitch, a suppressed gasp, a course of adrenalin.

Flush, heart-pound, tremble.

Do you feel the same?

How long have you been watching me?

The seal is perhaps four metres away. A common seal, a small one, young and puppy-like. Only the top of its head and muzzle are visible: dark reflective eyes you could drown in, converging nostrils. We make eye-contact. It sinks lazily and then dives, the arc of its back and its rear flippers briefly visible above the water.

I tread water and hold my breath, but not as long as the seal does.

There is no hint above the water of its whereabouts: I imagine it circling me, drifting through the tangles of Laminaria with occasional power-thrusts of its hind flippers, eyeing my pale, dangling limbs.

Whitworth goes on to examine what we know of the very different experience of a seal as it moves through water: how it senses the underwater world not only visually through its eyes but also via its vibrissae, sensory whiskers, which mean it can track an object moving through the water even when blindfolded.

She links that encounter, and the feelings she had, in the sea with this very other creature, to the sensation of *océanique* (a feeling that concerns the ocean), an idea discussed in the nineteenth century in letters between the French writer Romain Rolland – who believed it to be at the root of spiritual sentiment: a sense of limitlessness and of being at one with the external world – and Sigmund Freud.

Freud was at first resistant to the idea of *océanique*, but later would incorporate it into his theory, arguing, effectively, that as babies we start out in a state of oceanic consciousness, a feeling he locates within the primitive ego.

In her own dreamlike, attentive memoir, Whitworth writes:

If I experience the sensation océanique in the water does that mean I'm neurotic? In love, even? Can you fall in love with the sea, or with the seals? And I wonder whether my marriage would have been happier if my husband and I could have accepted each other as members of different species with alien but equally valid ways of engaging with the world. Can a seal understand echo-location, or an orca make sense of vibrissae?

I stay afloat, waiting for the sleek speckled head to re-emerge. When it does, the seal is much further away, perhaps twenty metres, heading westward. It looks over its shoulder at me one more time, then ducks again. This time it's for good. I wait nonetheless, still treading water. Slowly the dizzy, druggy sensation retreats, my heartbeat slows: I am back in my own skin, looking out through my own eyes.

In *Civilisation and its Discontents*, Freud described his correspondence with Rolland.

'A feeling as of something limitless, unbounded—as it were, "oceanic".'

Civilisation and its Discontents by Sigmund Freud[105]

I had sent [Rolland] my small book that treats religion as an illusion [*The Future of an Illusion* (1927)], and he answered that he entirely agreed with my judgement upon religion, but that he was sorry I had not properly appreciated the true source of religious sentiments. This, he says, consists in a peculiar feeling, which he himself is never without, which he finds confirmed by many others, and which he may suppose is present in millions of people. It is a feeling which he would like to call a sensation of 'eternity', a feeling as of something limitless, unbounded—as it were, 'oceanic'.

~

THE AUTHOR HERMANN HESSE WAS fascinated by Freud's ideas and was once voluntarily admitted to a mental hospital where he was psychoanalysed by Freud's one-time pupil, Carl Jung.

Hesse was a pacifist and a member of the anti-war movement in Germany during the First World War, and his wife, art historian Ninon Ausländer, was Jewish. He began his final novel, *The Glass Bead Game (Magister Ludi)* in 1931, when the Nazis were on the ascendant. It wasn't published until much later, in Switzerland, having been rejected by German publishers.

In it, the wise man Knecht has become a cloistered intellectual who plays a game with obscure rules. At one point he decides to take his wisdom and knowledge out into the world and tutor the young son of a friend, who embodies the Nazi ideal. But first, to show he is no mere bookworm, Knecht accepts the youth's invitation to a swimming race during which he suffers a heart attack and drowns. In some symbolic way, his death changes his pupil's consciousness.

"'If we swim very fast," he called out with boyish impetuosity, "we can just reach the other shore before the sun."'
The Glass Bead Game by Hermann Hesse[106]

In the morning, when Knecht sensed the house awakening, he rose. Finding a dressing gown laid ready beside his bed, he put it on, and stepped out. Before him the little lake lay motionless, gray-green. Further off was a steep cliff, its sharp, jagged crest still in shadow, rearing sheer and cold into the thin, greenish, cool morning sky. But he could sense that the sun had already risen behind this crest; tiny splinters of its light glittered here and there on corners of rock. In a few minutes the sun would appear over the crenellations of the mountain and flood lake and valley below with light.

Tito appeared, in bathing trunks. He shook hands with the Magister and pointing to the cliffs opposite said: 'You've come at just the right moment; the sun will be rising in a minute. Oh, it's glorious up here.'

Knecht gave him a friendly nod. He had learned long ago that Tito was an early riser, a runner, wrestler, and hiker, if only from protest against his father's casual, unsoldierly, comfort-loving ways. For the same reason he refused to drink wine. These leanings occasionally led him into a pose of being an anti-intellectual child of nature. But Knecht welcomed it all, and was determined to share his interest in sports as a means for winning over and taming the temperamental young man. It would be only one means among several, and not at all the most important; music, for example, would lead them much further. Of course he had no thought of matching the young man in physical feats, let alone surpassing him. But harmless participation would suffice to show the boy that his tutor was neither a coward nor a mere bookworm.

Tito looked eagerly toward the dark crest of the mountain, behind which the sky pulsed in the morning light. Now a fragment of the rocky ridge flashed violently like a glowing metal beginning to melt. The crest blurred and seemed suddenly lower, as if it were melting down, and from the fiery gap the dazzling sun appeared. Simultaneously, the ground, the house, and their shore of the lake were illuminated, and the two, standing in the strong radiance, instantly felt the delightful warmth of this light. The boy, filled with the solemn beauty of the moment and the glorious sensation of his youth and strength, stretched his limbs with rhythmic arm movements, which his whole body soon took up, celebrating the break of day in an enthusiastic dance and expressing his deep oneness with the surging, radiant elements. His steps flew in joyous homage toward the victorious sun and reverently retreated from it; his outspread arms embraced mountain, lake, and sky; kneeling, he seemed to pay tribute to the earth mother, and extending his hands, to the waters of the lake; he offered himself, his youth, his freedom, his burning sense of his own life, like a festive sacrifice to the powers. The sunlight gleamed on his tanned shoulders; his eyes were half-closed to the dazzle; his young face stared masklike with an expression of inspired, almost fanatical gravity. Without knowing what he was doing, asking no questions, he obeyed the command of this ecstatic moment, danced his worship, prayed to the sun, professed with devout movements and gestures his joy, his faith in life, his piety and reverence, both proudly and submissively offered up in the dance his devout soul as a sacrifice to the sun and the gods, and no less to the man he admired and feared, the sage and musician, the Master of the magic Game who had come to him from mysterious realms, his future teacher and friend.

All this, like the torrent of light from the sunrise, lasted only a few minutes. Stirred to the core, Knecht watched the wonderful show, in which his pupil before his eyes, changed and revealed himself, presenting himself in a new light, alien and entirely his equal. Both of them stood on the walkway, bathed in the radiance from the east and deeply shaken by their experience. Tito, having barely completed the last step of his dance, awoke from his ecstasy and stood still, like an animal surprised in solitary play, aware that he was not alone, that not only had he experienced and performed something unusual, but that he had also had a spectator. His first thought was how to extricate himself from the situation, which struck him now as somehow dangerous and shaming. He had to act vigorously, and smash the magic of these strange moments, which had totally absorbed and overwhelmed him. His face, but a moment before an ageless, stern mask, assumed a childish and rather foolish expression, like that of a person awakened too abruptly from a deep sleep. His knees swayed slightly; he looked into his teacher's face with vapid astonishment, and in sudden haste, as though something very important had just occurred to him, something he had neglected, he stretched out his right arm and pointed toward the opposite shore of the lake, which along with half the lake's waters still lay in the great, rapidly contracting shadow of the cliff whose top had already been conquered by the brilliance of the dawn.

'If we swim very fast,' he called out with boyish impetuosity, 'we can just reach the other shore before the sun.'

The words were barely uttered, the challenge to a swimming race with the sun barely issued, when Tito with a tremendous leap plunged headfirst into the lake, as if in his high spirits or his shyness he could not get away fast enough and obliterate all memory of the preceding ritual by intensified activity. The water splashed up and closed around him. A few moments later his head, shoulders, and arms reappeared and remained visible on the blue-green surface, swiftly moving away.

Knecht had not, when he came out, had in mind to bathe or swim. Both air and water were much too cool, and after his night of semi-illness, swimming would probably do him little good. But now, in the beautiful sunlight, stirred by the scene he had just witnessed, and with his pupil urging him into the water in this comradely fashion, he found the venture less deterring. Above all he feared that the promise born in this morning hour would be blasted if he disappointed the boy by opposing cool, adult rationality to this invitation to a test of strength. It was true that his feeling of weakness and uncertainty, incurred by the rapid ascent into the mountains, warned him to be careful; but perhaps this indisposition could be soonest routed by forcing matters and meeting it head-on. The summons was stronger than the warning, his will stronger than his instinct. He quickly shed the light dressing gown, took a deep breath, and threw himself into the water at the same spot where his pupil had dived.

The lake, fed by glacial waters so that even in the warmest days of summer one had to be inured to it, received him with an icy cold, slashing in its enmity. He had steeled himself for a thorough chilling, but not for this fierce cold which seemed to surround him with leaping flames and after a moment of fiery burning began to penetrate rapidly into him. After the dive he had risen quickly to the surface, caught sight of Tito swimming far ahead of him, felt bitterly assailed by this icy, wild, hostile element, but still believed he could lessen the distance, that he was engaging in the swimming race, was fighting for the boy's respect and comradeship, for his soul – when he was already fighting with Death, who had thrown him and was now holding him in a wrestler's grip. Fighting with all his strength, Knecht held him off as long as his heart continued to beat.

The young swimmer had looked back frequently and seen with satisfaction that the Magister had followed him into the water. Now he peered once again, no longer saw him, and became uneasy. Tito looked and called, then turned and swam rapidly back. He could not find him. Swimming and diving, he searched for the lost swimmer until his strength too began to give out in the bitter cold. Staggering, breathless, he reached land at last, saw the dressing gown lying on the shore, and picking it up began mechanically rubbing his body and limbs until the numbed skin warmed again. Stunned, he sat down in the sunlight and stared into the water, whose cool blue-green now blinked at him strangely empty, alien, and evil. He felt overpowered by perplexity and deep sorrow, for with the waning of his physical weakness, awareness and the terror of what had happened returned to him.

Oh! he thought in grief and horror, now I am guilty of his death. And only now, when there was no longer need to save his pride or offer resistance, he felt, in shock and sorrow, how dear this man had already become to him. And since in spite of all rational objections he felt responsible for the Master's death, there came over him, with a premonitory shudder of awe, a sense that this guilt would utterly change him and his life, and would demand much greater things of him than he had ever before demanded of himself.

CHAPTER II

The Sea as Mother

EACH YEAR ON 16 JUNE, Dublin celebrates *Ulysses* and James Joyce on 'Bloomsday', which begins with a dip at a swimming hole, the legendary Forty Foot. But it is not the only day on which its chill waters draw crowds. I've visited the turret-shadowed promontory quite a few times while researching books with my friend Anna, about swimming in Ireland. On the first occasion, the tide was high, with giant waves crashing in on the rocks and washing over the slippery paths. Though lifeguards still manned the box overlooking the water, all the swimmers had retreated to the adjacent shelter of Sandycove, overshadowed by the Martello tower where Joyce once lived. It thrummed with its regular dippers, like lively bird colonies perched along its wall, and seemed much the safer option.

Luckily, the next time I approached the Forty Foot, the sea was flat calm and I entered the water in the company of male mental-health swim group, the Blueballs. I remember standing at the top of the seaweed-fringed stairs leading down to that tight, rock-bound cove, and there must have been a man on every step. The millpond surface was shattered by the one-by-one, crashing entry of ecstatic bodies. The craic in the sea, as well as on the rocks, was of well-being, alcohol recovery and baring the soul, and what struck me then was how this bucket-list dip was a centre of community for so many in Dublin.

I also mused on the fact that, though for much of it history, and in Joyce's day, this was an all-male swimming spot, it is certainly no longer. Diving in straight after the Blueballs were the charismatic, laughter-exhaling all-female Dublin Dippers, and the following day, when I went back for more it was in the company of a women's group dedicated to the remarkable feat of swimming solely at sunrise all year round. Quite some challenge when, midsummer, it means setting an alarm for 3 a.m.! These days, it seems Joyce's 'scrotumtightening sea' is for all – whatever body parts we have for it to clasp its cold fingers around.

In the novel, the sea is linked in various ways with the main character Stephen Dedalus's mother. In this excerpt, Stephen is with 'stately, plump Buck Milligan' who frequently mocks both him and an English student, Haines, who is making a study of Irish customs.

'The snotgreen sea. The scrotumtightening sea.'
Ulysses by James Joyce[107]

Buck Mulligan wiped the razorblade neatly. Then, gazing over the handkerchief, he said:

—The bard's noserag! A new art colour for our Irish poets: snotgreen. You can almost taste it, can't you?

He mounted to the parapet again and gazed out over Dublin bay, his fair oakpale hair stirring slightly.

—God! he said quietly. Isn't the sea what Algy calls it: a great sweet mother? The snotgreen sea. The scrotumtightening sea. Epi oinopa ponton. Ah, Dedalus, the Greeks! I must teach you. You must read them in the original. Thalatta! Thalatta! She is our great sweet mother. Come and look.

Stephen stood up and went over to the parapet. Leaning on it he looked down on the water and on the mailboat clearing the harbourmouth of Kingstown . . .

—That reminds me, Haines said, rising, that I have to visit your national library today.

—Our swim first, Buck Mulligan said.

He turned to Stephen and asked blandly:

—Is this the day for your monthly wash, Kinch?

Then he said to Haines:

—The unclean bard makes a point of washing once a month.

—All Ireland is washed by the gulfstream, Stephen said as he let honey trickle over a slice of the loaf.

Haines from the corner where he was knotting easily a scarf about the loose collar of his tennis shirt spoke:

—I intend to make a collection of your sayings if you will let me . . .

He [Buck] capered before them down towards the fortyfoot hole, fluttering his winglike hands, leaping nimbly, Mercury's hat quivering in the fresh wind that bore back to them his brief birdsweet cries . . .

Two men stood at the verge of the cliff, watching: businessman, boatman.

—She's making for Bullock harbour.

The boatman nodded towards the north of the bay with some disdain.

—There's five fathoms out there, he said. It'll be swept up that way when the tide comes in about one. It's nine days today.

The man that was drowned. A sail veering about the blank bay waiting for a swollen bundle to bob up, roll over to the sun a puffy face, saltwhite. Here I am.

They followed the winding path down to the creek. Buck Mulligan stood on a stone, in shirtsleeves, his unclipped tie rippling over his shoulder. A young man clinging to a spur of rock near him, moved slowly frogwise his green legs in the deep jelly of the water.

—Is the brother with you, Malachi?

—Down in Westmeath. With the Bannons.

—Still there? I got a card from Bannon. Says he found a sweet young thing down there. Photo girl he calls her.

—Snapshot, eh? Brief exposure . . .

The young man shoved himself backward through the water and reached the middle of the creek in two long clean strokes. Haines sat down on a stone, smoking.

—Are you not coming in? Buck Mulligan asked.

—Later on, Haines said. Not on my breakfast.

Stephen turned away.

—I'm going, Mulligan, he said.

—Give us that key, Kinch, Buck Mulligan said, to keep my chemise flat.

Stephen handed him the key. Buck Mulligan laid it across his heaped clothes.

—And twopence, he said, for a pint. Throw it there.

Stephen threw two pennies on the soft heap. Dressing, undressing. Buck Mulligan erect, with joined hands before him, said solemnly:

—He who stealeth from the poor lendeth to the Lord. Thus spake Zarathustra.

His plump body plunged.

—We'll see you again, Haines said, turning as Stephen walked up the path and smiling at wild Irish.

Horn of a bull, hoof of a horse, smile of a Saxon.

—The Ship, Buck Mulligan cried. Half twelve.

—Good, Stephen said.

He walked along the upward-curving path.

Liliata rutilantium.

Turma circumdet.

Iubilantium te virginum.

The priest's grey nimbus in a niche where he dressed discreetly. I will not sleep here tonight. Home also I cannot go.

A voice, sweet-toned and sustained, called to him from the sea. Turning the curve he waved his hand. It called again. A sleek brown head, a seal's, far out on the water, round.

Usurper.

In the passage above, Buck Milligan refers to Algy, who calls the sea 'the great sweet mother'. This is a reference to the Victorian Pre-Raphaelite poet Algernon Charles Swinburne. Swinburne was fascinated by water and loved to immerse himself in rivers and the sea. He almost drowned at Étretat in Normandy when he was swept out by a strong tide – only to be rescued at the last minute by some fishermen.

'Mother and lover of men, the sea.'
'The Triumph of Time' by Algernon Charles Swinburne[108]

I will go back to the great sweet mother,
Mother and lover of men, the sea.
I will go down to her, I and none other,

Close with her, kiss her and mix her with me;
Cling to her, strive with her, hold her fast:
O fair white mother, in days long past
Born without sister, born without brother,
Set free my soul as thy soul is free.
O fair green-girdled mother of mine,
Sea, that art clothed with the sun and the rain,
Thy sweet hard kisses are strong like wine,
Thy large embraces are keen like pain.
Save me and hide me with all thy waves,
Find me one grave of thy thousand graves,
Those pure cold populous graves of thine
Wrought without hand in a world without stain.

~~~

IN HIS MEMOIR *The Lives of a Bengal Lancer*, Francis Yeats-Brown describes the river Ganges as a mother. Yeats-Brown, a distant relative of the poet W. B. Yeats, was a restless spirit whose writing offers a snapshot in time of what he observed about the customs of the country and the life of a colonial officer. Readers of Scottish writer Abir Mukherjee's popular series about the Raj era detective and opium addict Captain Sam Wyndham might trace a resemblance.

During the 1930s, Yeats-Brown fell to some degree under the sway of fascist ideas. But he signed up to serve in the British army in the Second World War when war broke out, in his fifties, and he was a serving officer at the time of his death in 1942.

'Then he submerges himself completely in the Mother.'

The Lives of a Bengal Lancer by Francis Yeats-Brown[109]

There is no sight more wonderful in all the world than the crescent-sweep of the Ganges on a bright morning, when Benares is at prayer. Three miles of crumbling palaces that lie in tumbled heaps with other palaces growing out of their ruins; and a confusion of richly-carved cupolas pushing their way between tamarind trees and tall flag-poles; and a fluttering of endless companies of pigeon among a forest of straw umbrellas; and below them a multitude of people who worship by the glittering water – peasants and priests, beggars and monstrosities, sacred bulls that have been married to four holy cows, cows with five legs, sleek girls with a skin of ivory and very poor and parched old women, fat merchants and thin fakirs, wise men and madmen, old and young, birds and beasts, all mingling on the bank and washing in the sacrosanct waters of the Mother – that is the river-front at Benares. The Ganges is so pure that you may drink beside her sewers, or amongst her corpses. She sprang from the feet of Vishnu, and from her was born the Hindu race. Her waters are jewels to the eyes of the living and sanctification to the parted lips of the dead. Her cult is ageless and casteless . . .

Yeats-Brown questions a guru.

Bhagawan Sri's pupils had returned for their evening lesson and were standing by the river steps, waiting to be called. Doves fluttered down from the palace ledges and flirted and bickered on the raft; a sacred bull stumbled down the steps and nosed the guru, as if wondering whether he was edible; and a fox terrier bitch appeared, brought by one of the pupils, wagging her tail and frisking round us.

'If I become a Yogi could I keep a dog?' I asked.

'Of course. Why not? She bathes with me every morning.'

'In the holy Ganges?'

'The Mother washes her as she washes me. The Ganges loves all our India, rich and poor, man and beast. There is nothing she cannot purify. We give to her the bodies of our dead and we drink her waters. That surprises you, but even your test-tubes tell you that we are right, for if you analyse the Ganges water you will find that it is Pure,'

'That is because it runs over such wide stretches of sand and beneath so much sunlight, guru-ji. But I do not question your views,' I hastened to add, 'I only ask to learn them.'

'Your feet have been led to the path. You have come here, and you will come again. To me, or to another, if I am dead. For you may not return for a long time.' Bhagawan Sri held out his hand . . . If you go to Benares, Sahib, you may find your guru. You may. I cannot tell. But I will give you his name, since I was told that you would come. It is Paramahansa Bhagawan Sri. Having humbled your heart and slain the desire of works, you may find him.'

They were slow, dreamy words, spoken not to me, it seemed, but to the Junma which was carrying down the white flowers and the yellow flowers that are the daily tribute of India to her gods and goddesses. Amongst these flowers rose an arm, as if waving a good-bye. It sank under the even waters, without sound or ripple, but the turtles had seen it and were coming from every direction, making tracks like the periscopes of submarines.

A big white turtle reached the body first, and worried it, and raised its obscene idiot's head with a ribbon of flesh in its mouth, snapping and gobbling. Others arrived. Soon there was a red foaming and scuffling where the body of a girl had been. I turned away, but Sivanand did not flinch.

CHAPTER III

Underworlds

IN THE WATER, SOMETIMES, PEOPLE dive deep and go to dark places. The journey takes us down and then back up again, to surface once more into the light, changed, perhaps, by what we found below. The sea in literature appears often as an underworld, an unsettling and ghostly realm for those of us who are its visitors.

These feelings haunt even descriptions of modern-day swimming such as the under-ice free dive performed by television presenter, Louise Minchin, in her 2023 book, *Fearless*.

'I pull myself under the ice and go for it.'
Fearless: Adventures with Extraordinary Women by Louise Minchin[110]

I look down into a triangle of pitch-black water in the centre of a frozen lake in Finland. It has been hacked out of ice a metre thick with a jagged saw. The surface looks oily and glutinous. It is as ominous and as featureless as a black hole in outer space. I am overwhelmed by a sense of fear and foreboding . . .

A Finnish woman is sitting on the edge next to me, dangling her feet, and she says to me: 'My theory on this is, just don't think about it. They have been overthinking it, just get on with it!'

I agree. My rational mind has taken over. I know I can hold my breath for at least a minute and a half. I know that with one breath and fins I can swim for at least 50 metres underwater. So, I know I can do this.

I make sure my lanyard is attached to the safety line, that my torch is working and that I can see through my mask. After a couple of deep breaths, I pull myself under the ice and go for it.

What happens next?

Massive sensory overload. *I am too buoyant. I am being squashed up against the underside of the ice so tightly that I can't swim. There is no air to breathe. It is dark, impossibly dark. I can't see the exit.* A switch clicks on in my brain and I go into survival mode. I am calm. *I can work this out.*

Time expands.

I turn onto my back, pressing my hand against the glassy underside of the ice, and push myself away so I can free my legs and kick. I register how surprisingly smooth it is. I thought it would be jagged, and my hands are telling me something different. I slide gracefully along, swimming on my back. I am suspended in space, floating without gravity. With my face turned towards the surface, I realise I can see the dim light of Cath's torch filtering through the thick ice, shining on me as she walks above my head. I focus on it and follow its tantalising beam as if it were a lifeline.

~

IN GREEK MYTHOLOGY, A DECEASED person's psyche or spirit would journey to the underworld by crossing the river Styx in a boat rowed by Charon, the ferry man. American writer John Cheever, sometimes called 'the Chekhov of the Suburbs' by Elmore Leonard, wrote elegant short stories of 'enchanted realism' in the mid-twentieth century. Neddy Merrill, the narrator of 'The Swimmer' – published in 1964 in *The New Yorker* – is at a drinks party in an affluent area of New York State when he works out that he can swim back to his home across the swimming pools of his well-heeled neighbours – a journey he calls 'The Lucinda River' after his wife.

But on the journey, the reader gradually realises that Neddy is in denial about the fact that he has lost his footing and no longer belongs to the class of the wealthy. He has been expelled from his paradise.

Pool owners react to him with pity or hostility. One says they are terribly sorry to hear of his misfortune, another is overheard telling someone that Neddy turned up drunk and tried to borrow $5,000. A former lover is rude to him and, when he reaches the end of his journey, the house, where he imagined his four beautiful daughters would be playing tennis, is locked up and empty. Dramatic and awash with undercurrents of sadness, some analysts have read 'The Swimmer' as a retelling of man's descent into the underworld.

'He had an inexplicable contempt for men who did not hurl themselves into pools.'

'The Swimmer' by John Cheever[111]

The day was beautiful and it seemed to him that a long swim might enlarge and celebrate its beauty. He took off a sweater that was hung over his shoulders and dove in. He had an inexplicable contempt for men who did not hurl themselves into pools. He swam a choppy crawl, breathing either with every stroke or every fourth stroke and counting somewhere well in the back of his mind the one-two one-two of a flutter kick. It was not a serviceable stroke for long distances but the domestication of swimming had saddled the sport with some customs and in his part of the world a crawl was customary. To be embraced and sustained by the light green water was less a pleasure, it seemed, than the resumption of a natural condition, and he would have liked to swim without trunks, but this was not possible, considering his project. He hoisted himself up on the far curb – he never used the ladder – and started across the lawn. When Lucinda asked where he was going he said he was going to swim home. The only maps and charts he had to go by were remembered or imaginary but these were clear enough. First there were the Grahams, the Hammers, the Lears, the Howlands, and the Crosscups . . .

The next pool on his list, the last but two, belonged to his old mistress Shirley Adams. If he had suffered any injuries at the Biswangers they would be cured here . . . They had had an affair last week, last month, last year. He couldn't remember. It was he who had broken it off, his was the upper hand, and he stepped through the gate of the wall that surrounded her pool with nothing so considered as self-confidence. It seemed in a way to be his pool . . . She was there, her hair the colour of brass, but her figure, at the edge of the lighted, cerulean water, excited in him no profound memories. It had been, he thought, a light-hearted affair, although she had wept when he broke it off. She seemed confused to see him and he wondered if she was still wounded. Would she, God forbid, weep again?

'What do you want?' She asked.

'I'm swimming across the county.'

'Good Christ. Will you ever grow up?'

'What's the matter?'

'If you've come here for money' she said, 'I won't give you another cent.'

'You could give me a drink.'

'I could but I won't. I'm not alone.'

'Well, I'm on my way.'

He dove in and swam the pool, but when he tried to haul himself up onto the curb he found that the strength in his arms and shoulders had gone, and he paddled to the ladder and climbed out. Looking over his shoulder he saw, in the lighted bathhouse, a young man. Going out onto the dark lawn he smelled chrysanthemums or marigolds – some stubborn autumnal fragrance – on the night air, strong as gas. Looking overhead he saw that the stars had come out, but why should he seem to see Andromeda, Cepheus, and Cassiopeia? What had become of the constellations of midsummer? He began to cry.

GERMAN ARCHAEOLOGIST LEO FROBENIUS coined the phrase 'The Night Sea Journey' to stand for all the stories when a hero finds himself (and it is usually a he) lost or drowning at sea, but is swallowed up by a sea monster or serpent inside whose belly he goes through a transformation, a kind of long, dark night of the soul.

For Carl Jung, the night sea journey was a metaphor for an exploration of the subconscious involving an encounter with one's suppressed fears. It carried, too, the danger of fracturing one's sense of self.

At school, I studied Joseph Conrad's 1910 tale of a ship's captain who, in the darkness of the night, comes across a man dangling at the bottom of the ladder cast outside his vessel. The initial image of the person clinging to the ladder out at sea was startling. He is a kind of phantom doppelganger, emerging from the underworld. This idea and the tale of an extraordinary swim stayed with me.

'Who'd have thought of finding a ladder hanging over at night in a ship anchored out here!'

'The Secret Sharer' by Joseph Conrad[112]

The riding light in the fore rigging burned with a clear, untroubled, as if symbolic, flame, confident and bright in the mysterious shades of the night. Passing on my way aft along the other side of the ship, I observed that the rope side ladder, put over, no doubt, for the master of the tug when he came to fetch away our letters, had not been hauled in as it should have been. I became annoyed at this, for exactitude in some small matters is the very soul of discipline. Then I reflected that I had myself peremptorily dismissed my officers from duty, and by my own act had prevented the anchor watch being formally set and things properly attended to. I asked myself whether it was wise ever to interfere with the established routine of duties even from the kindest of motives . . . I was vexed with myself.

Not from compunction certainly, but, as it were mechanically, I proceeded to get the ladder in myself. Now a side ladder of that sort is a light affair and comes in easily, yet my vigorous tug, which should have brought it flying on board, merely recoiled upon my body in a totally unexpected jerk. What the devil! . . . I was so astounded by the immovableness of that ladder that I remained stock-still, trying to account for it to myself like that imbecile mate of mine. In the end, of course, I put my head over the rail.

The side of the ship made an opaque belt of shadow on the darkling glassy shimmer of the sea. But I saw at once something elongated and pale floating very close to the ladder. Before I could form a guess a faint flash of phosphorescent light, which seemed to issue suddenly from the naked body of a man, flickered in the sleeping water with the elusive, silent play of summer lightning in a night sky. With a gasp I saw revealed to my stare a pair of feet, the long legs, a broad livid back immersed right up to the neck in a greenish cadaverous glow. One hand, awash, clutched the bottom rung of the ladder. He was complete but for the head. A headless corpse! The cigar dropped out of my gaping mouth with a tiny plop and a short hiss quite audible in the absolute stillness of all things under heaven. At that I suppose he raised up his face, a dimly pale oval in the shadow of the ship's side. But even then I could only barely make out down there the shape of his black-haired head. However, it was enough for the horrid, frost-bound sensation which had gripped me about the chest to pass off. The moment of vain exclamations was past, too. I only climbed on the spare spar and leaned over the rail as far as I could, to bring my eyes nearer to that mystery floating alongside.

As he hung by the ladder, like a resting swimmer, the sea lightning played about his limbs at every stir; and he appeared in it ghastly, silvery, fishlike. He remained as mute as a fish, too. He made no motion to get out of the water, either. It was inconceivable that he should not attempt to come on board, and strangely troubling to suspect that perhaps he did not want to. And my first words were prompted by just that troubled incertitude.

'What's the matter?' I asked in my ordinary tone, speaking down to the face upturned exactly under mine.

'Cramp,' it answered, no louder. Then slightly anxious, 'I say, no need to call anyone.

'I was not going to,' I said.

'Are you alone on deck?'

'Yes.'

I had somehow the impression that he was on the point of letting go the ladder to swim away beyond my ken—mysterious as he came. But, for the moment, this being appearing as if he had risen from the bottom of the sea (it was certainly the nearest land to the ship) wanted only to know the time. I told him. And he, down there, tentatively:

'I suppose your captain's turned in?'

'I am sure he isn't,' I said. He seemed to struggle with himself, for I heard something like the low, bitter murmur of doubt.

'What's the good?' His next words came out with a hesitating effort.

'Look here, my man. Could you call him out quietly?'

I thought the time had come to declare myself.

'I am the captain.'

I heard a 'By Jove!' whispered at the level of the water. The phosphorescence flashed in the swirl of the water all about his limbs, his other hand seized the ladder.

'My name's Leggatt.'

The voice was calm and resolute. A good voice. The self-possession of that man had somehow induced a corresponding state in myself. It was very quietly that I remarked:

'You must be a good swimmer.'

'Yes. I've been in the water practically since nine o'clock. The question for me now is whether I am to let go this ladder and go on swimming till I sink from exhaustion, or—to come on board here.'

I felt this was no mere formula of desperate speech, but a real alternative in the view of a strong soul. I should have gathered from this that he was young; indeed, it is only the young who are ever confronted by such clear issues. But at the time it was pure intuition on my part. A mysterious communication was established already between us two—in the face of that silent, darkened tropical sea. I was young, too; young enough to make no comment. The man in the water began suddenly to climb up the ladder, and I hastened away from the rail to fetch some clothes.

I got a sleeping suit out of my room and, coming back on deck, saw the naked man from the sea sitting on the main hatch, glimmering white in the darkness, his elbows on his knees and his head in his hands. In a moment he had concealed his damp body in a sleeping suit of the same gray-stripe pattern as the one I was wearing and followed me like my double on the poop. Together we moved right aft, barefooted, silent.

~

A LIGHTER TAKE ON THE night sea journey is found in the tale of Pinocchio. The Disney film was based on a late nineteenth-century Italian children's classic. Here a monstrous shark – known originally as 'The Terrible Dog-Fish' – swallows up the little puppet as he searches for his father Geppetto.

'Hey there, Mr. Fish, may I have a word with you?'
The Adventures of Pinocchio by Carlo Collodi[113]

Pinocchio saw a big Fish swimming near-by, with his head far out of the water.

Not knowing what to call him, the Marionette said to him: 'Hey there, Mr. Fish, may I have a word with you?'

'Even two, if you want,' answered the fish, who happened to be a very polite Dolphin.

'You who travel day and night through the sea, did you not perhaps meet a little boat with my father in it?'

'And who is your father?'

'He is the best father in the world, even as I am the worst son that can be found.'

'In the storm of last night,' answered the Dolphin, 'the little boat must have been swamped.'

'And my father?'

'By this time, he must have been swallowed by the Terrible Shark, which, for the last few days, has been bringing terror to these waters.'

'Is this Shark very big?' asked Pinocchio, who was beginning to tremble with fright.

'Is he big?' replied the Dolphin. 'Just to give you an idea of his size, let me tell you that he is larger than a five story building and that he has a mouth so big and so deep, that a whole train and engine could easily get into it.'

Pinocchio's heart beat fast, and then faster and faster. He redoubled his efforts and swam as hard as he could. Suddenly a horrible sea monster stuck its head out of the water, an enormous head with a huge mouth, wide open, showing three rows of gleaming teeth, the mere sight of which would have filled you with fear. Do you know what it was?

That sea monster was no other than the enormous Shark, which has often been mentioned in this story and which, on account of its cruelty, had been nicknamed 'The Attila of the Sea' by both fish and fishermen.

Poor Pinocchio! The sight of that monster frightened him almost to death! He tried to swim away from him, to change his path, to escape, but that immense mouth kept coming nearer and nearer.

Pinocchio swam faster and faster, and harder and harder.

The monster overtook him and the Marionette found himself in between the rows of gleaming white teeth. Only for a moment, however, for the Shark took a deep breath and, as he breathed, he drank in the Marionette as easily as he would have sucked an egg. Then he swallowed him so fast that Pinocchio, falling down into the body of the fish, lay stunned for a half hour.

When he recovered his senses the Marionette could not remember where he was. Around him all was darkness, a darkness so deep and so black that for a moment he thought he had put his head into an inkwell. He listened for a few moments and heard nothing. Once in a while a cold wind blew on his face. At first he could not understand where that wind was coming from, but after a while he understood that it came from the lungs of the monster. I forgot to tell you that the Shark was suffering from asthma, so that whenever he breathed a storm seemed to blow.

Pinocchio at first tried to be brave, but as soon as he became convinced that he was really and truly in the Shark's stomach, he burst into sobs and tears. 'Help! Help!' he cried. 'Oh, poor me! Won't someone come to save me?'

'Who is there to help you, unhappy boy?' said a rough voice, like a guitar out of tune.

'Who is talking?' asked Pinocchio, frozen with terror.

'It is I, a poor Tunny swallowed by the Shark at the same time as you. And what kind of a fish are you?'

'I have nothing to do with fishes. I am a Marionette.'

'If you are not a fish, why did you let this monster swallow you?'

'I didn't let him. He chased me and swallowed me without even a "by your leave"! And now what are we to do here in the dark?'

'Wait until the Shark has digested us both, I suppose.'

'But I don't want to be digested,' shouted Pinocchio, starting to sob.

'Neither do I,' said the Tunny, 'but I am wise enough to think that if one is born a fish, it is more dignified to die under the water than in the frying pan.'

'What nonsense!' cried Pinocchio.

'Mine is an opinion,' replied the Tunny, 'and opinions should be respected.'

'But I want to get out of this place. I want to escape.'

'Go, if you can!'

'Is this Shark that has swallowed us very long?' asked the Marionette.

'His body, not counting the tail, is almost a mile long.'

While talking in the darkness, Pinocchio thought he saw a faint light in the distance.

'What can that be?' he said to the Tunny.

'Some other poor fish, waiting as patiently as we to be digested by the Shark.'

'I want to see him. He may be an old fish and may know some way of escape.'

'I wish you all good luck, dear Marionette.'

'Goodbye, Tunny.'

'Goodbye, Marionette, and good luck.'

'When shall I see you again?'

'Who knows? It is better not to think about it.'

CHAPTER IV

The Power of Nature

FROM ACCIDENTS AT SEA TO disasters when a river breaks its banks – literature is full of illustrations of the powerlessness of little people against the immensity of water.

Herman Melville wrote his epic novel *Moby-Dick* in 1851. It stars the *Pequod*, a Nantucket whaling ship, whose multiracial crew is led by a madman obsessed with the great white whale. When crewman Pip jumps from the whaleboat out of panic, the second mate, Stubb, tells him that it is not worth losing a catch to rescue him because, if he were a slave, he would sell for a thirtieth of the price of a whale. But Pip jumps from the boat a second time and the trauma of being lost in the sea turns him into a kind of holy fool. In this liminal state, Pip becomes the only person who can connect with the terrifying Captain Ahab.

'He saw God's foot upon the treadle of the loom.'
Moby-Dick by Herman Melville[114]

'Stick to the boat, Pip, or by the Lord, I won't pick you up if you jump; mind that. We can't afford to lose whales by the likes of you; a whale would sell for thirty times what you would, Pip, in Alabama. Bear that in mind, and don't jump any more.'

But we are all in the hands of the Gods; and Pip jumped again. It was under very similar circumstances to the first performance; but this time he did not breast out the line; and hence, when the whale started to run, Pip was left behind on the sea, like a hurried traveller's trunk. Alas! Stubb was but too true to his word. It was a beautiful, bounteous, blue day; the spangled sea calm and cool, and flatly stretching away, all round, to the horizon, like gold-beater's skin hammered out to the extremest. Bobbing up and down in that sea, Pip's ebony head showed like a head of cloves. No boat-knife was lifted when he fell so rapidly astern. Stubb's inexorable back was turned upon him; and the whale was winged. In three minutes, a whole mile of shoreless ocean was between Pip and Stubb. Out from the centre of the sea, poor Pip turned his crisp, curling, black head to the sun, another lonely castaway, though the loftiest and the brightest.

Now, in calm weather, to swim in the open ocean is as easy to the practised swimmer as to ride in a spring-carriage ashore. But the awful lonesomeness is intolerable. The intense concentration of self in the middle of such a heartless immensity, my God! who can tell it? Mark, how when sailors in a dead calm bathe in the open sea — mark how closely they hug their ship and only coast along her sides.

But had Stubb really abandoned to his fate? No; he did not mean to, at least. Because there were two boats in his wake, and he supposed, no doubt, that they would of course come up to Pip very quickly, and pick him up . . . But it so happened, that those boats, without seeing Pip, suddenly spying whales close to them on one side, turned, and gave chase; and Stubb's boat was now so far away, and he and all his crew so intent upon his fish, that Pip's ringed horizon began to expand around him miserably. By the merest chance the ship itself at last rescued him; but from that hour the little negro went about the deck an idiot; such, at least, they said he was. The sea had jeeringly kept his finite body up, but drowned the infinite of his soul. Not drowned entirely, though. Rather carried down alive to wondrous depths, where strange shapes of the unwarped primal world glided to and fro before his passive eyes; and the miser-merman, Wisdom, revealed his hoarded heaps; and among the joyous, heartless, ever-juvenile eternities, Pip saw the multitudinous, God-omnipresent, coral insects, that out of the firmament of waters heaved the colossal orbs. He saw God's foot upon the treadle of the loom, and spoke it; and therefore his shipmates called him mad. So man's insanity is heaven's sense; and wandering from all mortal reason, man comes at last to that celestial thought, which, to reason, is absurd and frantic; and weal or woe, feels then uncompromised, indifferent as his God.

~

IN THIS APOCALYPTIC PASSAGE FROM *Their Eyes Were Watching God*, Zora Neale Hurston's 1937 classic of the Harlem Renaissance, her lead characters Janie and Tea Cake have to swim for their lives as they fight against what seems like an attack by an angry god when Lake Okeechobee in Florida floods. In fact, they refer to the noises of the storm as 'Ole Massa', as if God is a celestial slave-owner. Tea Cake kills a rabid dog which bites and infects him – and later in the narrative, Janie has to kill him.

'Their eyes straining against crude walls and their souls asking if He meant to measure their puny might against His.'
Their Eyes Were Watching God by Zora Neale Hurston[115]

Sometime that night the winds came back . . . when Janie looked out of her door she saw the drifting mists gathered in the west—that cloud field of the sky—to arm themselves with thunders and march forth against the world. Louder and higher and lower and wider the sound and motion spread, mounting, sinking, darking.

It woke up old Okechobee and the monster began to roll in his bed. Began to roll and complain like a peevish world on a grumble. The folks in the quarters and the people in the big houses further around the shore heard the big lake and wondered. The people felt uncomfortable but safe because there were the seawalls to chain the senseless monster in his bed. The folks let the people do the thinking. If the castles thought themselves secure, the cabins needn't worry. Their decision was already made as always. Chink up your cracks, shiver in your wet beds and wait on the mercy of the Lord. The bossman might have the thing stopped before morning anyway. It is so easy to be hopeful in the day time when you can see the things you wish on. But it was night, it stayed night. Night was striding across nothingness with the whole round world in his hands . . .

A big burst of thunder and lightning that trampled over the roof of the house. So Tea Cake and Motor stopped playing. Motor looked up in his angel-looking way and said, 'Big Massa draw him chair upstairs.'

'Ah'm glad y'all stop dat crap-shootin' even if it wasn't for money,' Janie said. 'Ole Massa is doin' His work now. Us oughta keep quiet.'

They huddled closer and stared at the door. They just didn't use another part of their bodies, and they didn't look at anything but the door. The time was past for asking the white folks what to look for through that door. Six eyes were questioning God.

Through the screaming wind they heard things crashing and things hurtling and dashing with unbelievable velocity. A baby rabbit, terror-ridden, squirmed through a hole in the floor and squatted off there in the shadows against the wall, seeming to know that nobody wanted its flesh at such a time. And the lake got madder and madder with only its dikes between them and him.

In a little wind-lull, Tea Cake touched Janie and said, 'Ah reckon you wish now you had of stayed in yo' big house 'way from such as dis, don't yuh?'

'Naw.'

'Naw?'

'Yeah, naw. People don't die till dey time come nohow, don't keer where you at. Ah'm wid mah husband in uh storm, dat's all.'

'Thanky, Ma'am. But 'sposing you wuz tuh die, now. You wouldn't git mad at me for draggin' yuh heah?'

'Naw. We been tuhgether round two years. If you kin see de light at daybreak, you don't keer if you die at dusk. It's so many people never seen de light at all. Ah wuz fumblin' round and God opened de door.'

He dropped to the floor and put his head in her lap. 'Well then, Janie, you meant whut you didn't say, 'cause Ah never knowed you wuz so satisfied wid me lak dat. Ah kinda thought—'

The wind came back with triple fury, and put out the light for the last time. They sat in company with the others in other shanties, their eyes straining against crude walls and their souls asking if He meant to measure their puny might against His. They seemed to be staring at the dark, but their eyes were watching God . . .

When the flood waters rise, Tea Cake and Janie leave their cabin on foot.

They stepped out in water almost to their buttocks and managed to turn east . . . Dodging flying missiles, floating dangers, avoiding stepping in holes and warmed on the wind now at their backs until they gained comparatively dry land. They had to fight to keep from being pushed the wrong way and to hold together. They saw other people like themselves struggling along. A house down, here and there, frightened cattle. But above all the drive of the wind and the water. And the lake. Under its multiplied roar could be heard a mighty sound of grinding rock and timber and a wail. They looked back. Saw people trying to run in raging waters and screaming when they found they couldn't. A huge barrier of the makings of the dike to which the cabins had been added was rolling and tumbling forward. Ten feet higher and as far as they could see the muttering wall advanced before the braced-up waters like a road crusher on a cosmic scale. The monstropolous beast had left his bed. The two hundred miles an hour wind had loosed his chains. He seized hold of his dikes and ran forward until he met the quarters; uprooted them like grass and rushed on after his supposed-to-be conquerors, rolling the dikes, rolling the houses, rolling the people in the houses along with other timbers. The sea was walking the earth with a heavy heel . . .

'De lake is comin'!' Tea Cake gasped.

'It's comin' behind us!' Janie shuddered. 'Us can't fly.'

'But we still kin run,' Tea Cake shouted and they ran. The gushing water ran faster. The great body was held back, but rivers spouted through fissures in the rolling wall and broke like day. The fugitives ran past another line of shanties that topped a slight rise and gained a little. They cried out as best they could, 'De lake is comin'!' and barred doors flew open and others joined them in flight crying the same as they went. 'De lake is comin'!' and the pursuing waters growled and shouted ahead, 'Yes, Ah'm comin'!', and those who could fled on . . .

The lake was coming on. Slower and wider, but coming. It had trampled on most of its supporting wall and lowered its front by spreading.

But it came muttering and grumbling onward like a tired mammoth just the same.

Tea Cake and Janie were some distance from the house before they struck serious water. Then they had to swim a distance, and Janie could not hold up more than a few strokes at a time, so Tea Cake bore her up till finally they hit a ridge that led on towards the fill. It seemed to him the wind was weakening a little so he kept looking for a place to rest and catch his breath. His wind was gone. Janie was tired and limping, but she had not had to do that hard swimming in the turbulent waters, so Tea Cake was much worse off. But they couldn't stop. Gaining the fill was something but it was no guarantee. The lake was coming. They had to reach the six-mile bridge. It was high and safe perhaps.

Everybody was walking the fill. Hurrying, dragging, falling, crying, calling out names hopefully and hopelessly. Wind and rain beating on old folks and beating on babies. Tea Cake stumbled once or twice in his weariness and Janie held him up. So they reached the bridge at Six Mile Bend and thought to rest. But it was crowded. White people had preempted that point of elevation and there was no more room. They could climb up one of its high sides and down the other, that was all. Miles further on, still no rest.

They passed a dead man in a sitting position on a hummock, entirely surrounded by wild animals and snakes. Common danger made common friends. Nothing sought a conquest over the other. Another man clung to a cypress tree on a tiny island. A tin roof of a building hung from the branches by electric wires and the wind swung it back and forth like a mighty ax. The man dared not move a step to his right lest this crushing blade split him open. He dared not step left for a large rattlesnake was stretched full length with his head in the wind. There was a strip of water between the island and the fill, and the man clung to the tree and cried for help.

'De snake won't bite yuh,' Tea Cake yelled to him. 'He skeered tuh go intuh uh coil. Skeered he'll be blowed away. Step round dat side and swim off!'

Soon after that Tea Cake felt he couldn't walk anymore. Not right away. So he stretched long side of the road to rest. Janie spread herself between him and the wind and he closed his eyes and let the tiredness seep out of his limbs. On each side of the fill was a great expanse of water like lakes—water full of things living and dead. Things that didn't belong in water. As far as the eye could reach, water and wind playing upon it in fury. A large piece of tar-paper roofing sailed through the air and scudded along the fill until it hung against a tree. Janie saw it with joy. That was the very thing to cover Tea Cake with. She could lean against it and hold it down. The wind wasn't quite so bad as it was anyway. The very thing. Poor Tea Cake!

She crept on hands and knees to the piece of roofing and caught hold of it by either side. Immediately the wind lifted both of them and she saw herself sailing off the fill to the right, out and out over the lashing water. She screamed terribly and released the roofing which sailed away as she plunged downward into the water.

'Tea Cake!' He heard her and sprang up. Janie was trying to swim but fighting water too hard. He saw a cow swimming slowly towards the fill in an oblique line. A massive-built dog was sitting on her shoulders and shivering and growling. The cow was approaching Janie. A few strokes would bring her there.

'Make it tuh de cow and grab hold of her tail! Don't use yo' feet. Jus' yo' hands is enough. Dat's right, come on!'

Janie achieved the tail of the cow and lifted her head up along the cow's rump, as far as she could above water. The cow sunk a little with the added load and thrashed a moment in terror. Thought she was being pulled down by a gator. Then she continued on. The dog stood up and growled like a lion, stiff-standing hackles, stiff muscles, teeth uncovered as he lashed up his fury for the charge. Tea Cake split the water like an otter, opening his knife as he dived. The dog raced down the backbone of the cow to the attack and Janie screamed and slipped far back on the tail of the cow, just out of reach of the dog's angry jaws. He wanted to plunge in after her but dreaded the water, somehow. Tea Cake rose out of the water at the cow's rump and seized the dog by the neck. But he was a powerful dog and Tea Cake was over-tired. So he didn't kill the dog with one stroke as he had intended. But the dog couldn't free himself either. They fought and somehow he managed to bite Tea Cake high up on his cheek-bone once. Then Tea Cake finished him and sent him to the bottom to stay there. The cow relieved of a great weight was landing on the fill with Janie before Tea Cake stroked in and crawled weakly upon the fill again.

CHAPTER V

Journey's End

EVENTUALLY, A RIVER FLOWS INTO the sea. We can evoke this as a metaphor for the journey of a human life, and in this final section writers use water to consider mortality.

I love the excerpt below, where Christopher Isherwood muses on the meaning of death. It bought me some comfort at a difficult time. During the period of putting together this book, my mother died at home in East Lothian, a week after suffering a haemorrhagic stroke. Although we were assured by the medical team that she was not in pain, her death seemed painfully slow. A friend dropped off some lilies in bud and in the sickroom I tried to watch not the clock but the flowers. On the day my mother died, I slept on a couch in her room and when I opened my eyes, the blooms had appeared. I took a few hours' respite and went for a swim from one of the beautiful sandy beaches nearby. Entering the chilly water – to my pelvis, then my belly button, then the final, full plunge into the waves, I thought of my mother letting go of her life, and of all the ways in which we were connected. Soon after I came out of the water, I got a call from my sister. She opened the front door to the carers and a soft breeze came through the hall – when she went back into the room, our mother was no more.

A Single Man is a novella by Christopher Isherwood, whose

tumultuous, novel of the 1930s, *Goodbye to Berlin*, inspired the musical *Cabaret*. The novella's story is told from the point of view of a middle-aged college professor George, sometime after the death of his long-term partner Jim. In small-town USA in the early 1960s, George is isolated from the community because of his homosexuality. He is also sexually frustrated and longs to meet another lover. One evening he goes to the bar where he first met Jim in what he describes as a freer era at the end of the Second World War. There he encounters one of his students, Kenny, who seems to have gone there in hopes of meeting him. In the bar, Kenny asks George about the benefits of experience and suggests they go for a night swim.

'The waters of the ocean are not really other than the waters of the pool.'
A Single Man by Christopher Isherwood[116]

'Let me tell you something Kenny . . . I haven't gotten wise on anything . . . In my opinion, I personally have gotten sillier and sillier and sillier – and that's a fact.'

'No kidding, Sir? You can't mean that! You mean, sillier than when you were young?'

'Much, much sillier.'

'I'll be darned. Then experience is no use at all? You're saying it might just as well not have happened?'

'No. I'm not saying that. I only mean, you can't use it. But if you don't try to – if you just realise it's there and you've got it – then it can be kind of marvelous.'

'Let's go swimming,' says Kenny abruptly, as if bored by the whole conversation.

'All right.'

Kenny throws his head right back and laughs wildly. 'Oh – that's terrific!'

'What's terrific?'

'It was a test. I thought you were bluffing, about being silly. So I said to myself, I'll suggest doing something wild, and if he objects – even if he hesitates – then I'll know it was all a bluff . . . You don't mind my telling you that, do you, Sir?'

'Why should I?'

'Oh, that's terrific!'

'Well, I'm not bluffing – so what are we waiting for? You weren't bluffing, were you?'

'Hell, no!'

They jump up, pay, run out of the bar and across the highway and Kenny vaults the railing and drops down, about eight feet, on to the beach. George, meanwhile, is clambering over the rail, a bit stiffly. Kenny looks up, his face still lit by the boardwalk lamps: 'Put your feet on my shoulders, Sir.' George does so, drunk-trustful, and Kenny, with the deftness of a ballet-dancer, supports him by ankles and calves, lowering him almost instantly to the sand. During the descent, their bodies rub against each other, briefly but roughly. The electric field of the dialogue is broken. Their relationship, whatever it now is, is no longer symbolic. They turn and begin to run toward the ocean.

Already, the lights seem far, far behind. They are bright but they cast no beams; perhaps they are shining on a layer of high fog. The waves ahead are barely visible. Their blackness is immensely cold and wet. Kenny is tearing off his clothes with wild whooping cries. The last remaining minim of George's caution is aware of the lights and the possibility of cruise-cars and cops, but he doesn't hesitate, he is no longer able to; this dash from the bar can only end in the water. He strips himself clumsily, tripping over his pants. Kenny, stark naked now, has plunged and is wading straight in, like a fearless native warrior, to attack the waves. The undertow is strong. George flounders for a while in a surge of stones. As he finally struggles through and feels sand under his feet, Kenny comes body-surfing out of the night and shoots past him without a glance; a water-creature absorbed in its element.

As for George, these waves are much too big for him. They seem truly tremendous, towering up, blackness unrolling itself out of blackness, mysteriously and awfully sparkling, then curling over in a thundering slap of foam which is sparked with phosphorus. George has sparks of it all over his body, and he laughs with delight to find himself bejewelled. Laughing, gasping, choking, he is too drunk to be afraid; the salt water he swallows seems intoxicating as whisky. From time to time, he catches tremendous glimpses of Kenny, arrowing down some toppling foam-precipice. Then, intent upon his own rites of purification, George staggers out once more, wide-open-armed, to receive the stunning baptism of the surf. Giving himself to it utterly, he washes away thought. speech, mood, desire, whole selves, entire lifetimes; again and again he returns, becoming always cleaner, freer, less. He is perfectly happy by himself; it's enough to know that Kenny and he are the sole sharers of the element. The waves and the night and the noise exist only for their play. Meanwhile, no more than two hundred yards distant, the lights shine from the shore and the cars flick past up and down the highway, flashing their long beams. On the dark hillsides you can see lamps in the windows of dry homes. The dry are going dryly to their dry beds. But George and Kenny are refugees from dryness; they have escaped across the border into the water-world, leaving their clothes behind them for a customs fee.

And now, suddenly, here is a great, an apocalyptically great wave. and George is way out, almost out of his depth, standing naked and tiny before its presence, under the lip of its roaring upheaval and the towering menace of its fall. He tries to dive through it – even now he feels no real fear – but instead he is caught and picked up, turned over and over and over, flapping and kicking toward a surface which may be either up or down or sideways, he no longer knows.

And now Kenny is dragging him out, groggy-legged. Kenny's hands are under George's armpits and he is laughing and saying like a Nanny, 'That's enough for now!' And George, still water-drunk, gasps, 'I'm all right,' and wants to go straight back into the water. But Kenny says, 'Well, I'm not – I'm cold,' and Nanny-like he towels George, with his own shirt, not George's, until George stops him because his back is sore. The Nanny-relationship is so convincing, at this moment, that George feels he could curl up and fall immediately asleep right here, shrunk to child-size within the safety of Kenny's bigness. Kenny's body seems to have grown gigantic since they left the water. Everything about him is larger than life; the white teeth of his grin, the wide dripping shoulders, the tall slim torso with its heavy-hung sex, and the long legs, now beginning to shiver. 'Can we go back to your place, Sir?' he asks.

The walk home sobers George up. By the time they reach the house, he no longer sees the two of them as wild water creatures but as an elderly professor with sodden hair bringing home an exceedingly wet student in the middle of the night. After an awkward conversation, Kenny leaves. George wakes to find he has been put to bed in his pyjamas. His mind is awash with sexual fantasy, then he falls asleep snoring – and dies. The novella has told us the story of his last day.

But is all of George altogether present here? Up the coast a few miles north, in a lava reef under the cliffs, there are a lot of rock pools. You can visit them when the tide is out. Each pool is separate and different, and you can, if you are fanciful, give them names – such as George, Charlotte, Kenny, Mrs Strunk. Just as George and the others are thought of, for convenience, as individual entities, so you may think of a rock pool as an entity; though, of course, it is not. The waters of its consciousness – so to speak – are swarming with hunted anxieties, grim-jawed greeds, dartingly vivid intuitions, old crusty-shelled rock-gripping obstinacies, deep-down protean sparkling undiscovered secrets, ominous organisms motioning mysteriously, perhaps warningly, toward the surface light. How can such a variety of creatures coexist at all? Because they have to. The rocks of the pool hold their world together. And, throughout the day of the ebb tide, they know no other. But that long day ends at last; yields to the night-time of the flood. And, just as the waters of the ocean come flooding, darkening over the pools, so over George and the others in sleep come the waters of that other ocean; that consciousness which is no one in particular but which contains everyone and everything, past, present and future, and extends unbroken beyond the uttermost stars. We may surely suppose that, in the darkness of the full flood, some of these creatures are lifted from their pools to drift far out over the deep waters. But do they ever bring back, when the daytime of the ebb returns, any kind of catch with them? Can they tell us, in any manner, about their journey? Is there, indeed, anything for them to tell – except that the waters of the ocean are not really other than the waters of the pool?

NATURE'S TIME IS FAR SLOWER and older than time counted by anxious, worried women, as T. S. Eliot reminds us, in the *Four Quartets*. The river is also a metaphor for the journey of life.

'The river is within us.'

'The Dry Salvages', *Four Quartets* by T. S. Eliot[117]

> I do not know much about gods; but I think that the river
> Is a strong brown god—sullen, untamed and intractable,
> Patient to some degree, at first recognised as a frontier;
> Useful, untrustworthy, as a conveyor of commerce;
> Then only a problem confronting the builder of bridges.
> The problem once solved, the brown god is almost forgotten
> By the dwellers in cities—ever, however, implacable.
> Keeping his seasons and rages, destroyer, reminder
> Of what men choose to forget. Unhonoured, unpropitiated
> By worshippers of the machine, but waiting, watching and waiting.
> His rhythm was present in the nursery bedroom,
> In the rank ailanthus of the April dooryard,
> In the smell of grapes on the autumn table,
> And the evening circle in the winter gaslight.
> The river is within us, the sea is all about us;
> The sea is the land's edge also, the granite
> Into which it reaches, the beaches where it tosses
> Its hints of earlier and other creation:
> The starfish, the horseshoe crab, the whale's backbone;
> The pools where it offers to our curiosity
> The more delicate algae and the sea anemone.
> It tosses up our losses, the torn seine,

The shattered lobsterpot, the broken oar
And the gear of foreign dead men. The sea has many voices,
Many gods and many voices.
The salt is on the briar rose,
The fog is in the fir trees.
The sea howl
And the sea yelp, are different voices
Often together heard: the whine in the rigging,
The menace and caress of wave that breaks on water,
The distant rote in the granite teeth,
And the wailing warning from the approaching headland
Are all sea voices, and the heaving groaner
Rounded homewards, and the seagull:
And under the oppression of the silent fog
The tolling bell
Measures time not our time, rung by the unhurried
Ground swell, a time
Older than the time of chronometers, older
Than time counted by anxious worried women
Lying awake, calculating the future,
Trying to unweave, unwind, unravel
And piece together the past and the future,
Between midnight and dawn, when the past is all deception,
The future futureless, before the morning watch
When time stops and time is never ending;
And the ground swell, that is and was from the beginning,
Clangs
The bell.

~

AT THE CENTRE OF ARUNDHATI Roy's debut novel, *The God of Small Things*, which won the Booker Prize in 1997, is the Meenachil. It is the flow of life, unstoppable, around which all momentous things in the narrative happen, and it links the two lovers, low-caste Velutha and high-caste Ammu.

In the final chapter, Velutha floats on his back down the river. This man who represents a connection with nature and the small things, who is indeed the God of Small Things, is drifting on the current towards a forbidden love. Death, birth, life as a river . . . All are present in this beautiful brief passage.

'When he saw her the detonation almost drowned him.'
The God of Small Things by Arundhati Roy[118]

Velutha floated on his back, looking up at the stars. His paralysed brother and one-eyed father had eaten the dinner he had cooked for them and were asleep. So he was free to lie in the river and drift slowly with the current. A log. A serene crocodile. Coconut trees bent into the river and watched him float by. Yellow bamboo wept. Small fish took coquettish liberties with him.

He flipped over and began to swim. Upstream. Against the current. He turned towards the bank for one last look, treading water, feeling foolish for having been so sure. So *certain*.

When he saw her the detonation almost drowned him. It took all his strength to stay afloat. He trod water, standing in the middle of a dark river.

She didn't see the knob of his head bobbing over the dark river. He could have been anything. A floating coconut. In any case she wasn't looking. Her head was buried in her arms.

He watched her. He took his time.

Had he known that he was about to enter a tunnel whose only egress was his own annihilation, would he have turned away?

Perhaps.

Perhaps not.

Who can tell?

OF COURSE, IT IS NOT only the river that brings us metaphors, lessons, even comforts. There is also, as we have shown previously, the ocean.

What the sea can teach us about change, grief and acceptance is touched on towards the end of Joan Didion's illuminating grief memoir, *The Year of Magical Thinking* – a slender book I read, between swims, as I travelled Ireland in the wake of my brother's death.

In the final lines of this account of her mind's journey over the year following the death of her husband, John, Didion recalls how – on around 'half a dozen' occasions –, she had gone swimming with him near a cave in California, and how they had to be in the water when the tide was just right.

In this excerpt, Didion uses the phrase 'no eye is on the sparrow', a reference to a classic hymn that asserts God's eye is on the sparrow. Didion did not believe in that eye. From childhood, Didion was awestruck by geological forces like earthquakes. She took comfort in their indifference: the indifference of nature to human needs and the lack of an overarching plan by an unknown being for her life.

'The tide had to be just right.'
The Year of Magical Thinking by Joan Didion[119]

I flew into Indonesia and Malaysia and Singapore with John, in 1979 and 1980. Some of the islands that were there then would now be gone, just shallows.

I think about swimming with him into the cave at Portuguese Bend, about the swell of clear water, the way it changed, the swiftness and power it gained as it narrowed through the rocks at the base of the point. The tide had to be just right. We had to be in the water at the very moment the tide was right. We could only have done this a half dozen times at most during the two years we lived there but it is what I remember. Each time we did it I was afraid of missing the swell, hanging back, timing it wrong. John never was. You had to feel the swell change. You had to go with the change. He told me that. No eye is on the sparrow but he did tell me that.

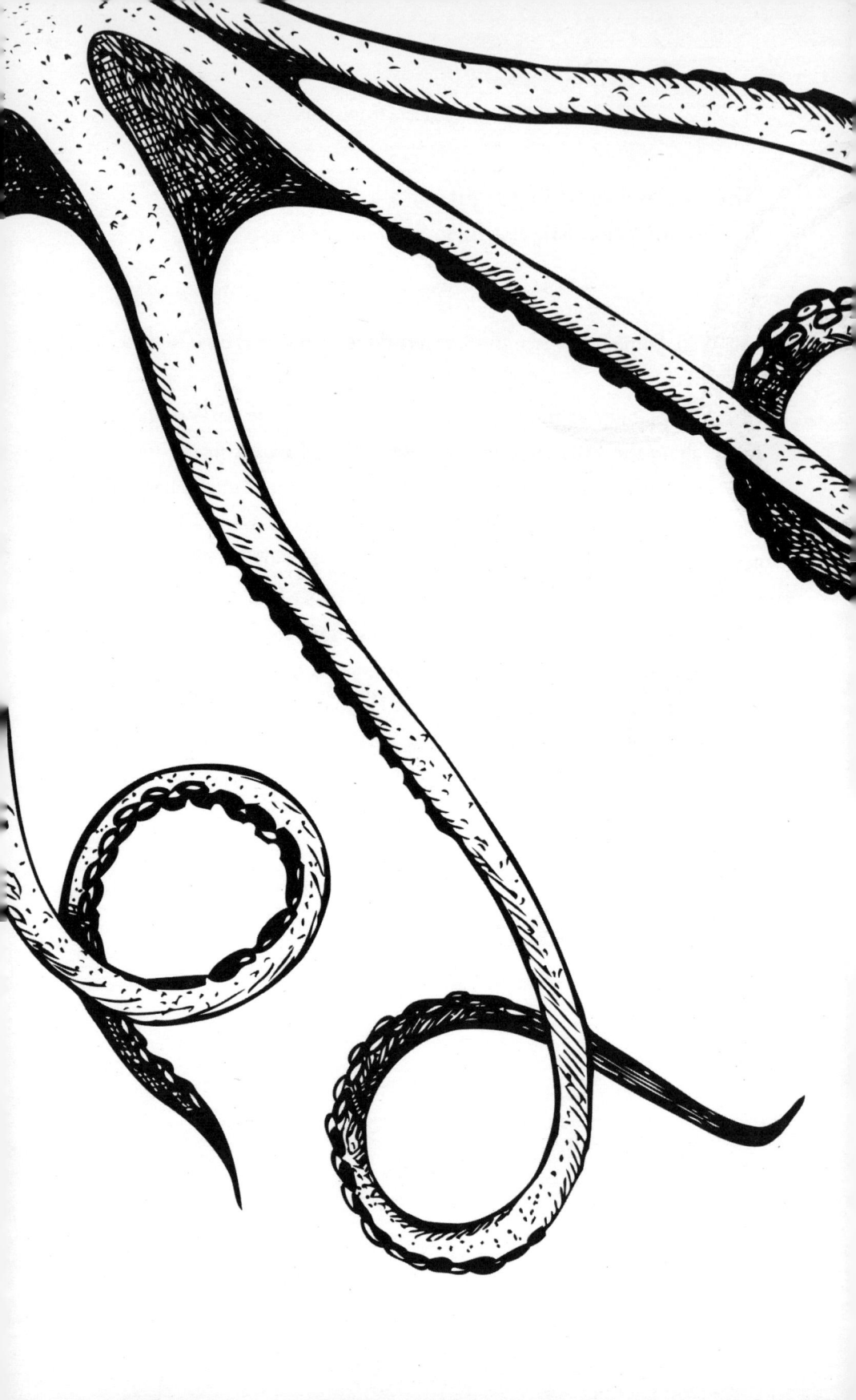

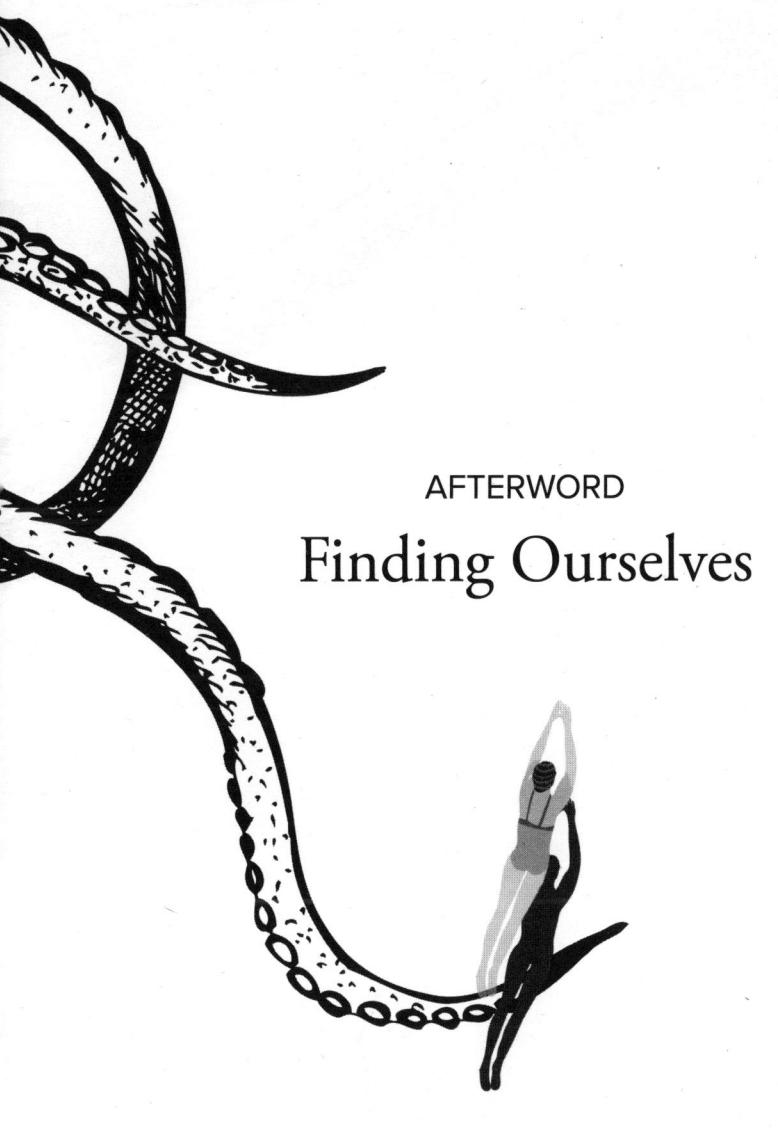

AFTERWORD

Finding Ourselves

'It's always ourselves we find in the sea.'

ONE OF THE THINGS WE often hear people say is that they 'found' themselves in swimming, retrieving some essential, sometimes lost self, a little bit of childhood, an almost-forgotten sense of play, or a connection to the big, wild, unjudging space of nature. The sea, for instance, is where Greystones swimmer and recovered alcoholic, Conor Brown, describes – in *Swimming Wild Ireland!* – a turning point in his recovery. 'I met me, I met Conor Brown,' he says simply.

There are, of course, other places in which we find ourselves – and books are one of them. Sometimes in their pages we get to 'meet me', as well as others whose words reach out and touch us. Bringing this anthology together has been a journey of 'aha' moments like these, of repeated recognition, in which we have found authors who perfectly expressed the feelings that we have had while swimming, who seem in some way to have travelled the very same waters as we have.

Sometimes, they are our contemporaries; sometimes their swims are centuries distant. But it can feel as if we share the same watery world, the same fear and wonder.

Books are one of the places we go to find connection and know others; where, perhaps, we do not feel so alone. That, too, reminds us of swimming, and of the shoreside communities who through plunging as a group so often generate that sense of togetherness. The water is a space in which people can connect with each other and also with something that feels much bigger.

While we have worked on this book, we have kept up our own rhythms of dipping, mostly in the seas off Scotland, sometimes apart, sometimes together, as we holed up in a cottage above chill but inviting Loch Torridon. It has been a shared space – the tidal estuary between words and water.

We hope you have enjoyed sharing it with us and felt some of those same intakes of breath, chuckles of recognition, and the occasional 'aha'.

From early on, we had a feeling that there was one poem we wanted to end on, which chimed with our own experience of the sea as both a childhood pleasure and a joyful dissolving of self. It's a short verse rich with moments of mutual understandings, much loved the world over. And, naturally, it touches on what exactly it is we find in the sea.

'maggie and milly and molly and may
went down to the beach (to play one day)
and maggie discovered a shell that sang
so sweetly she couldn't remember her troubles, and
milly befriended a stranded star
whose rays five languid fingers were;
and molly was chased by a horrible thing
which raced sideways while blowing bubbles: and
may came home with a smooth round stone
as small as a world and as large as alone.
For whatever we lose (like a you or a me)
it's always ourselves we find in the sea'

— E. E. CUMMINGS,
maggie and milly and molly and may[120]

Reading List

EPIGRAPH

[1] *The Living Mountain* by Nan Shepherd (1977)

The Living Mountain © Nan Shepard 1977. Reproduced with permission of the Licensor through PLSclear.

AN OCEAN OF WORDS

[2]'Swimming, One Day in August' by Mary Oliver (2008)

Reprinted by the permission of The Charlotte Sheedy Literary Agency as agent for the author. Copyright © 2008 by Mary Oliver with permission of Bill Reichblum.

Play: Swimming and Childhood

I: SUMMER HOLIDAYS

[3] *Swallows and Amazons* by Arthur Ransome (1930)

From *Swallows and Amazons* by Arthur Ransome published by Red Fox. Copyright © Arthur Ransome, 1930. Reprinted by permission of The Random House Group Limited.

[4] *The Summer Book* by Tove Jansson (1974)

From *The Summer Book* translated from Swedish by Thomas Teal in 1974. This translation is reproduced here with permission from Sort of Books.

[5]'Memory Laps' by David Sedaris (2011)

'Memory Laps' by David Sedaris published in *The New Yorker*, 2011.

[6] *Made in Scotland: My Grand Adventures in a Wee Country* by Billy Connolly (2018)

From *Made In Scotland* by Billy Connolly published by Vintage. Copyright © Billy Connolly, 2018. Reprinted by permission of The Random House Group Limited.

[7] *A Vicarage Family* by Noel Streatfeild (2016)

From *A Vicarage Family* by Noel Streatfeild published by Puffin. Copyright © Noel Streatfeild, 2016. Reprinted by permission of Penguin Books Limited.

[8] 'At the Bay' by Katherine Mansfield (1922)

II: SWIMMING LESSONS

[9] *The Story of My Boyhood and Youth* by John Muir (1913)

[10] *A Question of Climate* by Audre Lorde (1986)

I Am Your Sister: Collected and Unpublished Writings of Audre Lorde © Oxford University Press, Inc. 2009. Reproduced with permission of the Licensor through PLSclear.

[11] *The Lady and the Sharks* by Eugenie Clark (2010)

The Lady and the Sharks © Eugenie Clark 2010. Reproduced with permission of the Peppertree Press, LLC.

[12] 'Letters and Papers on Philosophical Subjects' in *The Works of Benjamin Franklin* by Jared Sparks (editor) (1856)

III: THE RIGHT TO SWIM

[13] 'Big Boy Leaves Home' by Richard Wright (1936)

Reprinted by permission of John Hawkins and Associates, Inc. Copyright © 1936, 1937, 1938 by Richard Wright, Restored edition copyright 1999 by Julia Wright.

[14] *Uncle Tom's Cabin* by Harriet Beecher Stowe (1852)

[15] *Huckleberry Finn* by Mark Twain (1884)

IV: PARENTS ON THE EDGE

[16] 'The Winter Father' by Andre Dubus (1980)

Andre Dubus, excerpts from 'The Winter Father' from *The Winter Father*. Copyright © 1980 by Andre Dubus. Reprinted with the permission of The Permissions Company, LLC on behalf of David R Godine, Publisher, Inc., godine.com.

[17] *Anna Karenina* by Leo Tolstoy (1878)

[18] *Letter to My Father* by Franz Kafka (1919)

[19] *A House for Mr Biswas* by V. S. Naipaul (1961)

A House for Mr Biswas by V. S. Naipaul. Copyright © 1961, V. S. Naipaul, used by permission of The Wylie Agency (UK) Limited.

V: ADVENTURE

[20] *A Prayer for Owen Meany* by John Irving (1989)

From *A Prayer for Owen Meany* by John Irving published by Black Swan. Copyright © John Irving, 1989. Reprinted by permission of The Random House Group Limited.

[21] *John Macnab* by John Buchan (1928)

[22] *Little House on the Prairie* by Laura Ingalls Wilder (1935)

Reprinted by permission of HarperCollins Publishers Ltd. © 1935 Laura Ingalls Wilder.

[23] *Kidnapped* by Robert Louis Stevenson (1886)

VI: ADULTS AT PLAY

[24] 'Out to Play', from *Taking the Plunge* by Vicky Allan and Anna Deacon (2019)

[25] *Three Men in a Boat* by Jerome K. Jerome (1889)

[26] 'The Kanaka Surf' by Jack London (1917)

Scary: Monsters and Marvels

I: SEE MONSTERS

[27] *The Sea, The Sea* by Iris Murdoch (1978)

From *The Sea, The Sea* by Iris Murdoch published by Vintage Classics. Copyright © Iris Murdoch, 1978. Reprinted by permission of The Random House Group Limited.

[28] *Beowulf*, translated by John Lesslie Hall (1892)

[29] 'The Diver' by Friedrich Schiller (1798)

[30] *Alice's Adventures in Wonderland* by Lewis Carroll (1863)

II: MARVELLOUS SEA CREATURES

[31]*A Gift to Those Who Contemplate the Wonders of Cities and the Marvels of Travelling* by Ibn Battuta (1355)

[32]*Fasti*, Book II by Ovid (43 BC–17 AD)

Ovid. *Fasti*. Translated by Frazer, James George. Loeb Classical Library Volume. Cambridge, MA, Harvard University Press; London, William Heinemann Ltd. 1931.

[33]*Songs of Maldoror* by the Comte de Lautréamont (1868)

III: MONSTERS ARE US

[34]*Sule Skerry*, Orkney ballad (1850s)

[35]*The Selkie that Deud No' Forget* by Walter Traill Dennison (1880)

[36]'A Man Young and Old: III. The Mermaid' from *The Tower* by W. B. Yeats (1928)

[37]*The Sea Lady* by H. G. Wells (1901)

[38]*Small Bodies of Water* by Nina Mingya Powles (2021)

Small Bodies of Water © Nina Mingya Powles 2021. Reproduced with permission of the Licensor through PLSclear.

[39]*The Descent of Woman* by Elaine Morgan (1972)

The Descent of Woman © Elaine Morgan 1972. Reprinted with permission of Souvenir Press.

Sensation: Swimming and desire

I: FEELING WATER

[40]'Where Ice Meets Fluidity', from *Taking the Plunge* by Vicky Allan and Anna Deacon (2019)

[41]*The Living Mountain* by Nan Shepherd (1977)

The Living Mountain © Nan Shepard 1977. Reproduced with permission of the Licensor through PLSclear.

[42]'Song of Myself' by Walt Whitman (1885)

[43]'I started Early – Took my Dog' by Emily Dickinson (from *Poems*) (1891)

[44]'On Swimming', in *Mediterranean Inspiration* by Paul Valéry (1933)

II: EROTIC ENCOUNTERS

[45]*The Sharing Economy* by Sophie Berrebi (2023)

The Sharing Economy © Sophie Berrebi 2023. Reprinted with permission of Simon & Schuster.

[46]'Frieda and Lawrence' by David Garnett, in *D. H. Lawrence: Novelist, Poet, Prophet* (edited by Stephen Spender) (1973)

'Frieda and Lawrence' © David Garnett 1973. Reprinted with permission of United Agents.

[47]*Women in Love* by D. H. Lawrence (1920)

[48]*The Awakening* by Kate Chopin (1899)

[49]'Charmides' by Oscar Wilde (1881)

[50]'Song of Myself' by Walt Whitman (1885)

[51]*The Swimming-Pool Library* by Alan Hollinghurst (1988)

From *The Swimming-Pool Library* by Alan Hollinghurst published by Vintage. Copyright © Alan Hollinghurst, 1988. Reprinted by permission of The Random House Group Limited.

[52]'A Bather' by Amy Lowell (1917)

III: OLD TIMES

[53]'The Book of the Thousand Nights and a Night', *A Plain and Literal Translation of the Arabian Nights Entertainments* by Richard Francis Burton (1888)

[54]*Marcus Antonius, Plutarch's Lives* (translated from Greek by Aubrey Stewart and George Long) (1892)

IV: THE MALE GAZE

[55]'Gooseberries' by Anton Chekhov (1898)

[56]*The Duel* by Anton Chekhov (1891)

[57]'The Swimmers' by F. Scott Fitzgerald (1929)

V: SEXY BEASTS

[58] 'The Water-Nymph' by Alexander Pushkin (1819)

VI: FREE FROM THE GAZE

[59] *I Found My Tribe* by Ruth Fitzmaurice (2018)

I Found My Tribe by Ruth Fitzmaurice. Published by Chatto & Windus. Copyright © Ruth Fitzmaurice, 2018. Reprinted by permission of The Random House Group Limited.

[60]'An open letter to every plus-size swimmer who's afraid of being mocked at the pool' by Ella Foote (2019)

Reprinted by permission of Ella Foote.

Epic: Great Swims

I: COLD WATERS, COLD WARS

[61]'A World of Difference' by Lewis Pugh (2021)

Reprinted by permission of Lewis Pugh.

[62] *Swimming to Antarctica* by Lynne Cox (2004)

Excerpt from *Swimming to Antarctica: Tales of a Long Distance Swimmer* by Lynne Cox, copyright © 2004 by Lynne Cox. Used by permission of Lynne Cox.

[63] *The Private Life of Chairman Mao* by Dr Li Zhisui (1996)

From *The Private Life of Chairman Mao* by Zhisui Li published by Chatto & Windus. Copyright © Zhisui Li, 1996. Reprinted by permission of The Random House Group Limited.

[64]Letter from John F. Kennedy to Inga Arvad (1965)

The material included in the John F. Kennedy Personal Papers was donated to the Kennedy Library in 1965.

[65]Handwritten note by John F. Kennedy, JFK Presidential Library (1965)

The material included in the John F. Kennedy Personal Papers was donated to the Kennedy Library in 1965.

II: STRONG SWIMMERS

[66] *Shifting Currents: A World History of Swimming* by Karen Carr (2022)

Shifting Currents: A World History of Swimming © Karen Carr 2022.

[67] *Twelve Years a Slave* by Solomon Northrup (1853)

[68] *The Art of Swimming* by Melchisédech Thévenot (1696)

[69] *A Gift to Those Who Contemplate the Wonders of Cities and the Marvels of Travelling* by Ibn Battuta (1355)

[70] *Why We Swim* by Bonnie Tsui (2020)

From *Why We Swim* by Bonnie Tsui published by Rider. Copyright © Bonnie Tsui, 2020. Reprinted by permission of The Random House Group Limited.

III: ANCIENTS

[71] *The Odyssey* by Homer (800 BCE)

[72] 'Poseidon' from *North Sea Song* by Heinrich Heine (1825)

[73] 'Conduct of Cloelia', *The History of Rome* by Livy (1919)

[74] *The Lays of Ancient Rome* by Thomas Barrington Macaulay (1860)

IV: ALONGSIDE SWIM HEROES

[75] *Written After Swimming from Sestos to Abydos* by Lord Byron (1810)

[76] 'Tarry, delight, so seldom met' by A. E. Housman (1936)

[77] *Pōkarekare Ana* (1914)

[78] *The Count of Monte Cristo* by Alexandre Dumas (1846)

V: LOST

[79] *Historia de Expeditione Frederici Imperatoris* (1827)

[80] 'Lycidas' by John Milton (1637)

[81] Note on Poems of 1822 by Mrs. Shelley (1839)

[82] 'A Shropshire Lad' by John Betjeman (2003)

A Shropshire Lad' from *Best Loved Poems of John Betjeman* by John Betjeman (2003). Reproduced with permission of the Licensor through PLSclear.

Well: The Cold Water Cure

I: RECOVERY

[83] *I Found My Tribe* by Ruth Fitzmaurice (2018)

I Found My Tribe by Ruth Fitzmaurice. Published by Chatto & Windus. Copyright © Ruth Fitzmaurice, 2018. Reprinted by permission of The Random House Group Limited.

[84] *The Outrun* by Amy Liptrot (2017)

The Outrun © Amy Liptrot 2017. Reproduced with permission of the Licensor through PLSclear.

[85] *The Ripple Effect* by Anna Deacon and Vicky Allan (2023)

[86] *The Tidal Year* by Freya Bromley (2023)

The Tidal Year © Freya Bromley 2023. Reproduced with permission of the Licensor through PLSclear.

II: THE DOCTOR'S LINE

[87] *The Life of Charlemagne* by Einhard (1880)

[88] *A Short introduction for to learne to Swimme* by Everard Digby (1595)

[89] *Psychrolousia. Or, The History of Cold Bathing* by John Floyer (1697)

[90] *Burns From a New Point of View* by James Crichton-Browne (1925)

III: TAKING THE WATERS

[91] *The Expedition of Humphry Clinker* by Tobias Smollett (1771)

[92] Queen Victoria's journal, Friday 30 July 1847

[93] *Sanditon* by Jane Austen (1817)

[94] A letter from Jane Austen to her sister Cassandra, from Lyme, September 1804

[95] *The Life of Charlotte Brontë* by Elizabeth Gaskell (1857)

IV: LITERALLY WILD

[96] *Walden* by Henry David Thoreau (1854)

[97] The George Sand–Gustave Flaubert Letters, translated by Aimee L. McKenzie (1921)

V: REDISCOVERY

[98] *Waterlog* by Roger Deakin (1999)

Waterlog by Roger Deakin published by Vintage. Copyright © Roger Deakin, 1999. Reprinted by permission of The Random House Group Limited.

[99] *Pondlife: A Swimmer's Journal* by Al Alvarez (2013)

Pondlife: A Swimmer's Journal © Al Alvarez, 2013.

[100] *Turning: Lessons from Swimming Berlin's Lakes* by Jessica J. Lee (2018)

Turning: A Swimming Memoir © Jessica J. Lee 2018. Reproduced with permission of the Licensor through PLSclear.

Deep: Swimming and Symbolism

I: OCÉANIQUE

[101] *Swimming Wild Ireland!* by Anna Deacon and Vicky Allan (2024)

[102] *Gilead* by Marilynne Robinson (2004)

Gilead © Marilynne Robinson 2004. Reproduced with permission of the Licensor through PLSclear.

[103] *The Interpretation of Dreams* by Sigmund Freud (1899)

[104] *Swimming with Seals* by Victoria Whitworth (2017)

Swimming with Seals © Victoria Whitworth 2017. Reproduced with permission of Bloomsbury Sport, an imprint of Bloomsbury Publishing Plc.

[105] *Civilisation and its Discontents* by Sigmund Freud (1930)

[106] *The Glass Bead Game* by Hermann Hesse (1943)

From *The Glass Bead Game* by Hermann Hesse published by Jonathan Cape. Copyright © Herman Hesse, 1943. Reprinted by permission of The Random House Group Limited.

II: THE SEA AS MOTHER

[107] *Ulysses* by James Joyce (1920)

[108]'The Triumph of Time' by Algernon Charles Swinburne (1866)

[109] *The Lives of a Bengal Lancer* by Francis Yeats-Brown (1930)

III: UNDERWORLDS

[110] *Fearless: Adventures with Extraordinary Women* by Louise Minchin (2023)

Fearless: Adventures with Extraordinary Women © Louise Minchin 2023. Reproduced with permission of Bloomsbury Sport, an imprint of Bloomsbury Publishing Plc.

[111]'The Swimmer' by John Cheever (1964)

From *Collected Stories* by John Cheever published by Jonathan Cape. Copyright © John Cheever, 1964. Reprinted by permission of The Random House Group Limited.

[112]'The Secret Sharer' by Joseph Conrad (1910)

[113] *The Adventures of Pinocchio* by Carlo Collodi (1883)

IV: THE POWER OF NATURE

[114] *Moby-Dick* by Herman Melville (1851)

[115] *Their Eyes Were Watching God* by Zora Neale Hurston (1937)

Their Eyes Were Watching God © Zora Neale Hurston 1937. Reproduced with permission of the Licensor through PLSclear.

V: JOURNEY'S END

[116] *A Single Man* by Christopher Isherwood (1964)

From *A Single Man* by Christopher Isherwood published by Vintage Classics. Copyright © Christopher Isherwood, 1964. Reprinted by permission of The Random House Group Limited.

[117]'The Dry Salvages', *Four Quartets* by T. S. Eliot (1941)

'The Dry Salvages', *Four Quartets* © T. S. Eliot 1941. Reproduced with permission of Faber and Faber Ltd.

[118] *The God of Small Things* by Arundhati Roy (1997)

The God of Small Things © Arundhati Roy 1997. Reproduced with permission of the Licensor through PLSclear.

[119] *The Year of Magical Thinking* by Joan Didion (2006)

Reprinted by permission of HarperCollins Publishers Ltd © 2006 Joan Didion.

AFTERWORD: FINDING OURSELVES

[120] *maggie and milly and molly and may: A Poem* by E. E. Cummings (1956)

'maggie and milly and molly and may'. Copyright © 1956, 1984, 1991 by the Trustees for the E. E. Cummings Trust, from *COMPLETE POEMS: 1904-1962* by E. E. Cummings, edited by George J. Firmage. Used by permission of Liveright Publishing Corporation.

Acknowledgements

Thank you to the National Library of Scotland where we have read and re-read many half-remembered books in the course of researching this collection. Thanks to the friendly and helpful staff.

Thanks also to the team at Black & White, the many publishers we have contacted to arrange copyright permission and to the writers who have allowed us to use their material. Thanks, in particular, to our editor Emma Hargrave.

Lastly, thanks to our families and friends for their support and interest in this project and for their helpful suggestions.

Jackie and Vicky